look better naked!

Editor-in-Chief of Women's Health
Michele Promaulayko
with Maura Rhodes

look better naked!

Editor-in-Chief of Women's Health
Michele Promaulayko

with Maura Rhodes

photography by Ondrea Barbe

RODALE®

Notice

The information in this book is meant to supplement, not replace, proper exercise training. All forms of exercise pose some inherent risks. The editors and publisher advise readers to take full responsibility for their safety and know their limits. Before practicing the exercises in this book, be sure that your equipment is well-maintained, and do not take risks beyond your level of experience, aptitude, training, and fitness. The exercise and dietary programs in this book are not intended as a substitute for any exercise routine or dietary regimen that may have been prescribed by your doctor. As with all exercise and dietary programs, you should get your doctor's approval before beginning. Mention of specific companies, organizations, or authorities in this book does not imply endorsement by the author or publisher, nor does mention of specific companies, organizations, or authorities imply that they endorse this book, its author, or the publisher. Internet addresses and telephone numbers given in this book were accurate at the time it went to press.

Rodale books may be purchased for business or promotional use or for special sales. For information, please write to: Special Markets Department, Rodale Inc., 733 Third Avenue, New York, NY 10017

Women's Health is a registered trademark of Rodale Inc.

Printed in the United States of America
Rodale Inc. makes every effort to use acid-free ♾, recycled paper ♻.

Photographs by Ondrea Barbe

Book design by Davia deCroix with George Karabotsos,
design director of Men's Health Books and Women's Health Books

Dust jacket cover by Lan Yin Bachelis

For complete list of credits, please see page 293.

Library of Congress Cataloging-in-Pulication Data is on file with the publisher.

ISBN-10: 1-60529-463-2
ISBN-13: 978-1-60529-463-6

Distributed to the trade by Macmillan

2 4 6 8 10 9 7 5 3 1 hardcover

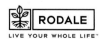

We inspire and enable people to improve their lives and the world around them
For more of our products visit **rodalestore.com** or call 800-848-4735

This book is for every woman who
has ever cringed a little while stripping off
the camouflage we call clothes—
in the bedroom, bathroom, or locker room.
You deserve to have complete
in-the-buff confidence, and I'm going
to help you get it!

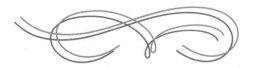

contents

acknowledgments

Look Better Naked is my first book as the editor-in-chief of *Women's Health*, but it wouldn't be in your hands without some incredibly hard-working people. I'd like to take this opportunity to thank them.

First and foremost is Maura Rhodes, my co-author, who did everything beautifully and in record time—all while moving into a new home and sending her oldest son away to college.

Next I'd like to thank the members of the Rodale family, especially our CEO and chairman, Maria, who helms this unique and reader-dedicated company. It's an honor to be here. On that note, I certainly wouldn't be editor-in-chief of *Women's Health*—my absolute dream job!—if it weren't for David Zinczenko, the magazine's editorial director, the senior vice president and editor-in-chief of *Men's Health*, and the bestselling author of *The Abs Diet* and the *Eat This, Not That!* book series. Dave, your drive and talent inspire me every day.

I'd also like to recognize Stephen Perrine and Debbie McHugh of *Men's Health* for their guidance. And Joel Weber for his brilliant conceptualizing and editing—you're an absolute gem! *Women's Health* contributors Rachel Cosgrove and Keri Glassman for creating the fitness and nutrition components; George Karabotsos and Davia deCroix for designing such a visually arresting book; Karen Rinaldi, EVP, general manager and publisher, Rodale Books, and Gregg Michaelson, president, integrated marketing and sales, chief marketing officer, for their tremendous efforts; Chris Krogermeier, Erin Williams, Brooke Myers, and Jodi Schaffer on the Rodale book team for shepherding *Look Better Naked* through its production; *Women's Health* creative director Andrea Dunham, deputy art director Lan Yin Bachelis, and photo director Sarah Rozen; photographers Ondrea Barbe (ondreabarbe.com) and Beth Bischoff; models Aline Fernandes and Melissa Re; Robert Lyons, Asami Taguchi, Nausil Zaheer, Manny Norena, Dan Ownes, Michiko Boorberg, Lauren Saldutti, and Thea Palad—all of whom helped coordinate demanding photo shoots; videographer Gunnar Waldman and personal trainer Jessica Smith for their contributions to the companion workout DVD; and Allison Keane, in advance, for her efforts to promote this book. I owe you all a huge debt of gratitude.

Last but not least, I'd like to thank all the journalists, editors, copy editors, researchers, designers, photographers, illustrators, Web producers, doctors, personal trainers, advisors, nutritionists, and others who have worked tirelessly in the past few years to build *Women's Health* into the world-class brand that it is today.

Michele Promaulayko

introduction

the naked truth

Naked.

Does any word cut so close to the core of our deepest insecurities? When we're naked, it's not just our bodies that are on exhibit—it's our hearts, our souls, our very self-worth that feels exposed and ripe for criticism. And if you're like most women, you know that no one can be as hard on you as well, you.

As the editor-in-chief of *Women's Health,* I hear from women every single day who share their greatest fears and their deepest anxieties about their bodies. And invariably, those stem from one thing: how they look naked.

That's why this book is for you: If you've ever looked in a mirror at your naked self and felt anything other than spectacular, then you've come to the right place. *Look Better Naked* is for women who want to look hotter, live healthier, and—perhaps most important of all—feel more confident, in clothes or out of them.

What I tell the millions of readers of *Women's Health* looking to achieve that goal is simple: I know exactly how you feel. Because many times, I've felt the very same way. And I've never been more intensely insecure about my body—and how it's changed over the years—than in the weeks and months leading up to my recent 20th high school reunion.

At the end of my senior year at Bridgewater High School in New Jersey, receiving a "senior superlative" award during our graduation dinner was almost as important as getting a diploma—at least in my teenage mind. I knew I shouldn't take the awards too seriously, that they were goofy titles, but I couldn't help myself. I secretly rested my hopes on being singled out for *something*. MOST LIKELY TO SUCCEED was out of reach, but maybe BEST ALL AROUND was in the cards—after all, I'd played varsity soccer, was on student council, and socialized with geeks, jocks, and partyers alike.

As I pushed roasted chicken around my plate to calm my nerves, our class president announced the first few awards. Thunderous applause met each winner's name, and the cheers grew louder and louder with each recognition. As I'd hoped, my closest friends were raking in the accolades. BEST LOOKING went to Betsy, Nicole easily nabbed SEXIEST, and my Broadway-bound pal Jeanine snagged MOST TALENTED. Then our class president made an announcement that I'm certain made my parents very proud: "And BEST BUNS goes to Michele Promaulayko!"

Evidently the Class of 1988 found my snug Guess jeans more memorable than my performance in the classroom or on the soccer field. I eventually forgave them (most of them, anyway), but by the time my 20-year reunion rolled around two decades later, I felt like my trophy behind had lost its star appeal. Sure, I'd put time and effort into trying to stave off gravity and stay in shape through the years, but I certainly wasn't twisting my neck to take notes on how my backside had "developed" as I'd gotten older, busier, and a little more complacent about the nutritional value of every morsel that passed my lips. Truth be told, I couldn't even remember the last time I'd caught a glimpse of my own bare bottom. I always wrapped in a towel before stepping out of the shower, I purposely dressed away from my full-length mirror, and I shopped online to avoid dressing rooms. As silly as hiding from my own naked reflection sounds, that sort of behavior wasn't unique or some temporary lapse of reason—it's commonplace among women today. One recent medical survey revealed that a mere 19 percent of women are happy with their bodies. In other words, of your five closest friends, only one of them thinks her physique deserves a thumbs-up. I'd love to say this figure surprises me, but it doesn't.

A nude body shows who we truly are physically—and too often we're not proud of our status. When we're naked and unadorned, we're totally vulnerable, exposing the workouts we've skipped and the high-cal desserts we've polished off. When we do find ourselves totally naked—maybe a couple of times a day, for a total of about 20 minutes—the unveiling usually happens because we're either showering or having sex, or somewhere between the two. Soon afterward many of us rush to swathe ourselves in a bedsheet or robe before finally hiding beneath our clothes—the armor we use to protect ourselves from the world. And, probably like you, I have spent years and a good chunk of money curating a wardrobe of brands that flatter my body (thank you, Diane von Furstenberg!) and silhouettes that act like the fashion equivalent of smoke and mirrors—highlighting assets and deflecting eyes away from the flagging trophies.

77% of women say that they're highly motivated to look better naked.

But I've found a way to escape that cycle of embarrassment—and to stop shying away from the mirror. A few months after my reunion (confession: I wore Spanx), I made the biggest career move of my life. I left a long-term stint at *Cosmopolitan* to become editor-in-chief of *Women's Health*—a magazine that serves up comprehensive (and sane!) advice on staying fit, healthy, and happy. And as I was getting to know the editorial staff as well as my colleagues at *Men's Health*, our brother magazine, what impressed me the most was their vast knowledge about the human body. To help readers achieve their fitness, weight-loss, and nutrition goals, they scour the latest studies in prestigious journals, interview dozens of the country's top experts, and, most important, practice what they preach—in the gym, in the kitchen, even in the office (where staffers regularly used the in-house yoga studio). They're health aficionados through and through, and their dedication to their craft show—in their flat stomachs and toned arms. I immediately knew that I'd come to the right place for getting my body back in peak condition.

But I also knew that I wasn't the only woman in America who was self-conscious about her naked body. So I surveyed more than 3,500 *Women's Health* readers for their thoughts. Seventy-two percent of them immediately said they looked better clothed than naked. And when I asked which body parts made them most self-conscious, 62 percent said their bellies, 22 percent said their butts, and 16 percent said their breasts. But then came the most important part: Some 77 percent said they were *highly motivated* for *Women's Health* to help them look better naked. So I got to work on this book.

Look Better Naked is an invitation to stop hiding from yourself, to rediscover—and reshape—the body beneath your clothes, and to boost your in-the-buff confidence. The next time you're about to step into the shower, take a look at your reflection in the mirror and stash the image in your memory bank. That's the last you're going to see of the old you. Then put aside the weight-loss and shape-up disappointments you've faced in the past and get ready to *look better naked*!

Michele

Michele Promaulayko

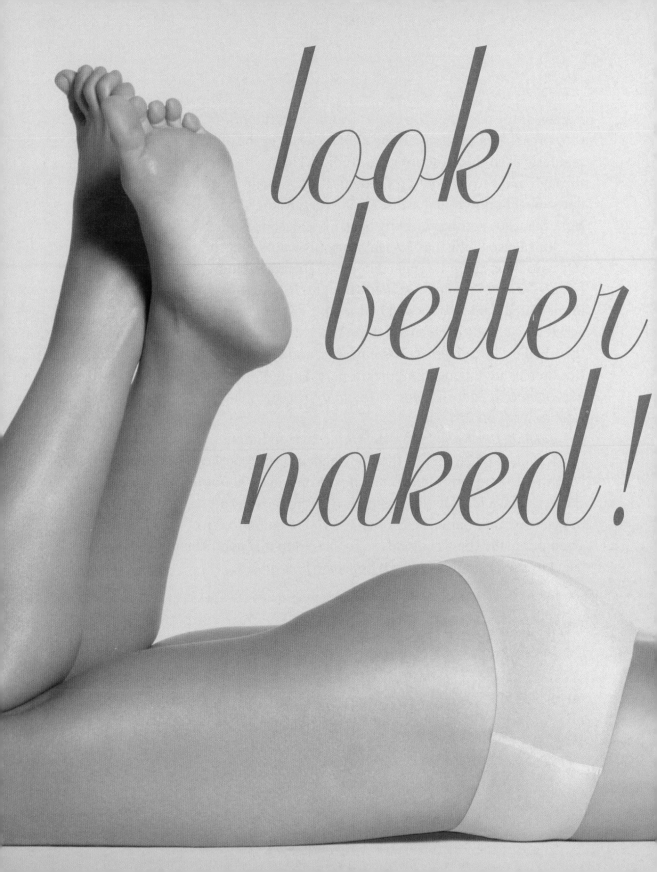

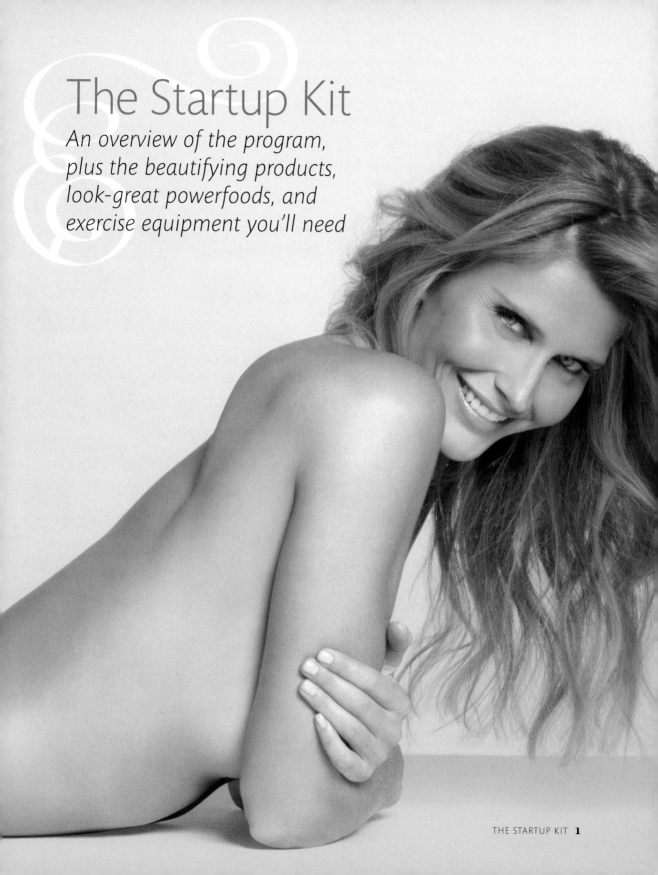

The Startup Kit

An overview of the program, plus the beautifying products, look-great powerfoods, and exercise equipment you'll need

overview

the diet

Kick-Start Strategy: A 2-day clean-food cleanse

Five Meals a Day: Breakfast, lunch, dinner, and two snacks

Magic Number: 1,400 calories daily

Secret Weapons: No- and low-calorie flavor-boosting spices, marinades, dressings, and condiments

Cheating: Occasional splurges to keep you grounded

Drinking: Unlimited green tea, water, and fat-free milk; occasional smoothies; and two glasses of wine or the signature Look Better Naked cocktail per week

Important Nutritional Components:
• Fiber-rich starches and fruits (at least 3 grams of fiber per serving)
• Lean protein (no more than 5 grams of fat per serving)
• Healthy fats (mono- and polyunsaturated)

the fitness plan

Exercise Program: Half "featherweight" strength training, half metabolism-boosting interval training

Commitment: Four days a week, 2 hours and change

Progression: New full-body workouts every 3 weeks

Timeline: Minimum 6 weeks

the extras

Special Treats: Massages, candlelight dinners, lingerie shopping, and bubble baths

Grooming Guidelines: How-to's for shaving, waxing, moisturizing, and more

your day at a glance

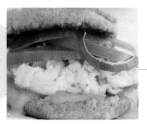

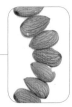

Begin with a breakfast that fuels your body—and your brain!

Snack twice a day to conquer your cravings!

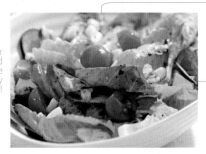

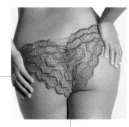

Eat power lunches and overcome midday energy crashes!

Shop for a sexy number that will accentuate your assets!

Feast on fat-fighting meals that will make you lean for life!

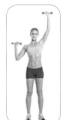

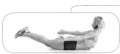

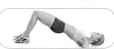

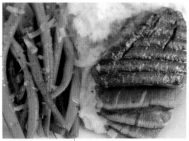

Hit the gym for one of your four weekly workouts!

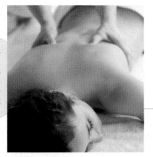

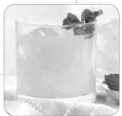

Finish your day with an intimate massage—and see where your night goes!

Out on the town? Order your new go-to cocktail.

pantry

Stock your shelves, fridge, and freezer with healthy and delicious fare. Some options:

the 20 LBN powerfoods

Avocados
Beef
Bell peppers
Berries
Black beans
Brussels sprouts
Cheese
Chicken breast
Dried fruit
Eggs
Flaxseed
Hummus
Milk
Nuts and nut butters
Olives and extra-virgin olive oil
Salmon
Tofu
Tuna
Whole-grains
Yogurt

staples

Apples
Artichokes
Asparagus
Beets
Broccoli
Cantaloupe
Carrots
Cauliflower
Celery
Cucumber
Edamame
Eggplant
Grapefruit
Halibut
High-fiber crackers
Leafy greens
Pineapple
Popcorn
Scallops
Shrimp
Squash
Sweet potatoes
Tilapia
Veggie burgers
Whole-wheat breads and pasta
Zucchini

flavor boosters

Barbecue sauce
Chutney
Cocoa powder
Dijon mustard
Dried spices (any, such as basil, cinnamon, oregano)
Fat-free cottage cheese
Fat-free, low-sodium chicken broth
Fresh ginger
Fresh herbs
Garlic
Guacamole
Honey
Hot pepper flakes
Ketchup
Lemon juice
Lime juice
Low-sodium soy sauce
Marinara sauce
Pepper
Salsa
Shredded coconut
Vinegars (balsamic, red wine, flavored)
White horseradish
Worcestershire sauce

tools

You truly won't need much "stuff" for this program, but here's what I recommend that you have access to.

gym membership

If you don't already belong to a gym, you should seriously consider joining one—even if only for the next 2 months. (Learn how to get a deal on page 100.) But if you're adamantly opposed to that option and are willing to improvise, you can get by with the following equipment:

- Adjustable bench
- Barbell and a few 5- and 10-pound plates
- Dumbbells, two or three pairs ranging from 5 to 20 pounds
- Exercise mat
- Jump rope
- Running shoes
- Swiss ball

beauty products

- Acne-clearing products
- Antibacterial body wash
- Body lotion
- Bronzer stick
- Cellulite-fighting cream
- Exfoliating scrub
- Facial moisturizer
- Full-body mirror
- Hair removal cream
- Self-tanner
- Waxing strips

cooking equipment

- Baking sheet
- Blender
- Cast-iron skillet
- Salad dressing shaker (optional but recommended)
- Stainless steel pot
- Toaster oven (optional but recommended)
- Vegetable steamer

what look better naked will do for you

Prepare to become firmer, fitter, healthier, and happier

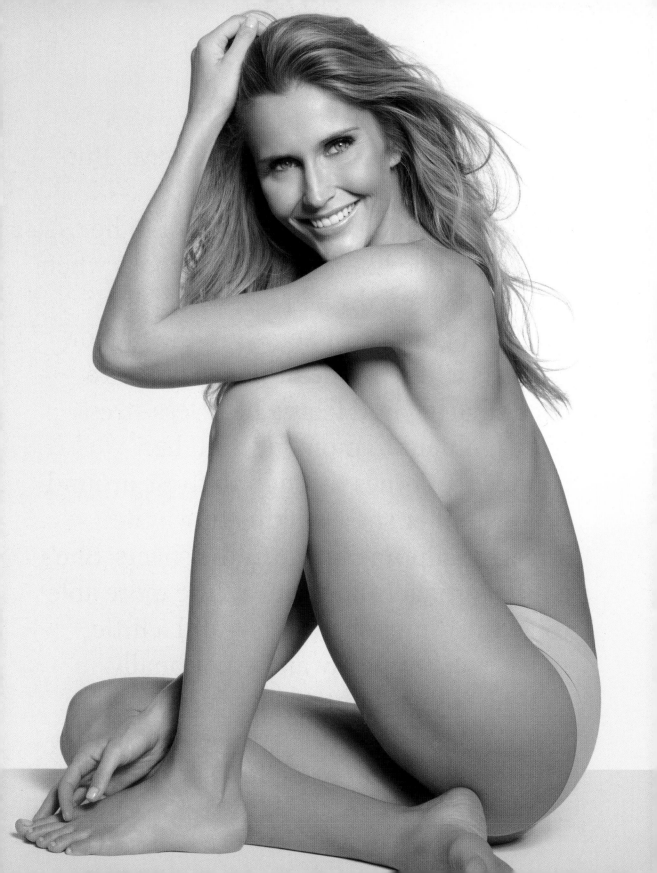

There's a woman out there somewhere who's a lot like you, in so many ways. But she's just a little bit . . . better.

She's a little bit more confident in her own skin: She likes the way she looks when she steps out of the shower, when she catches a glimpse of herself in the mirror. She eats a little bit healthier, exercises a little smarter, and feels a little less stress from moment to moment. And her confidence shines through to those around her—whether she's walking down the street, or slipping between the sheets. She's a little stronger than you, a little more able to do the things she wants—and a little more free, physically and emotionally.

Who *is* this slightly better version of you? Well, of course, it's you—the you that can and will be, in just a few short weeks.

You see, this book contains a complete plan for upgrading each and every aspect of your physical appearance. And it will help you alter your thinking about how you look, so you can welcome those physical changes, appreciate just how elastic and dynamic your physique truly is, and feel confident that you have ultimate control over your body. That may sound like a tall order, but it's one you're going to achieve by eating great food, never feeling tired or hungry, and discovering just how doable it is—and how little time it takes—to sculpt your best body ever.

You'll accomplish that without a fad diet, or a brutal workout program, or some intensive meditation plan. I'll teach you to eat better, to use short bursts of exercise to turbocharge your metabolism, and to change the ways you regard food, fitness, and your physical form. But a major reason *Look Better Naked* is different from other diet and workout books is that it takes into consideration the entire person that you are: a thinking, feeling, highly unique human being whose brain and body are connected. You can't *look* better naked unless you *feel* better naked, and vice versa.

This book will get you there.

Here's a sneak peek at what else you should expect to gain (or lose!) in the coming days, and how this book will change your life for the better.

50%
of women say that they spend less than 10 minutes au natural daily!

You'll Exude More Confidence!

Psychologists call the vision of yourself in your mind's eye body image. As the researchers who study the subject continue to discover, how we feel about our own bodies is *completely* subjective. When asked, women of all shapes, sizes, and ages routinely say that they're significantly larger than they actually are. As a result, the goal of looking and feeling your best seems further away than it actually is! You have the ability to improve your body image all by yourself—no shrink's couch required. Our mental make-over, designed to help you shed negative naked-self perceptions and build up your nude-body confidence, begins in just a few pages. Use it to eliminate your body-bashing mindset and begin to embrace the significant physical changes you're just weeks away from realizing!

You'll Have a Hotter Sex Life!

More than 50 percent of American adults have sex just once a week. Considering all the feel-good orgasms we're collectively missing out on, that's a seriously depressing thought. If you're part of the unlucky half, I want you to prepare to switch over to the pleasure-seeking side. Shying away from sex because you're self-conscious about stripping down will no longer be an issue, once you discover how to hang up your hang-ups. Instead, you'll be

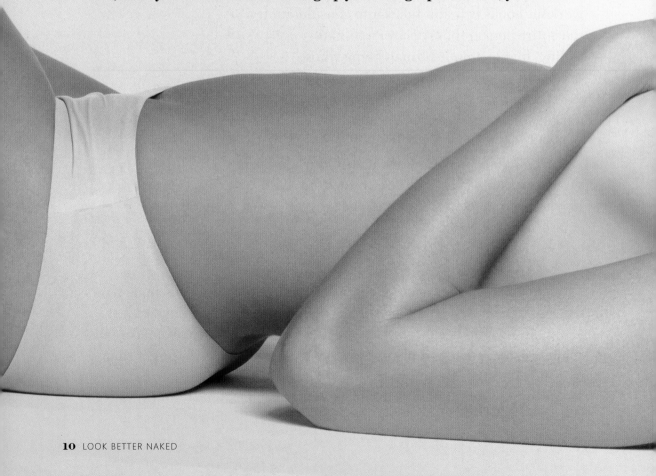

looking and feeling sexier, and having steamier sex—and lots more of it.

And if you're already getting it on with regularity? An additional boost of confidence will help turn good sex into great sex. Building your ego, it turns out, also stokes your libido. In a study published in the journal *Archives of Sexual Behavior,* women with higher levels of self-confidence about their bodies reported greater sexual desire than their sex-starved peers.

You'll Flatten Your Belly!

Two-thirds of American adults are now overweight, and the obesity rate has increased by nearly 50 percent in the past 50 years. It's a particular concern for the women I surveyed, 60 percent of whom said their bellies needed the most attention of all their body parts.

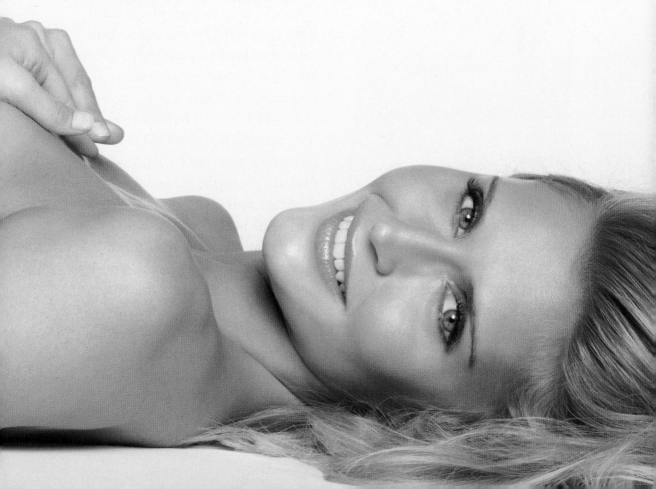

Well, here's some science that ought to give you pause—and hope! Belly fat is composed mostly of a type of tissue called visceral fat—that means fat that's hanging around your internal organs, pushing out your tummy. That's the most dangerous type of fat you can own—it's been linked to heart disease, diabetes, and more. But here's the good news: It's also the easiest type of fat to get rid of!

The key is to rev up your metabolism and stop sabotaging yourself with unhealthy meals. I know, I know—you try to eat healthy. We all do. But most of us don't realize how out of control our portion sizes have become. Even relatively healthy foods have become caloric catastrophes, and much of the extra weight we pack on is no fault of our own! Take spaghetti, for example. Four ounces of pasta—what nutritionists consider "one serving"—contains 422 calories. That's a modest meal in most cases. But how large is 4 ounces? When you hold the dried pasta together and view it from the end, it's about the diameter of a quarter! And if you think the cooks and chefs in restaurant kitchens are using that measurement, think again. The typical entrée at eateries such as the Olive Garden pack an average of 905 calories, and that doesn't include appetizers, drinks, sides, or desserts.

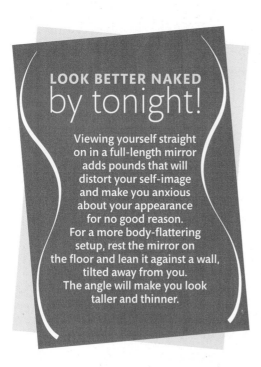

LOOK BETTER NAKED
by tonight!

Viewing yourself straight on in a full-length mirror adds pounds that will distort your self-image and make you anxious about your appearance for no good reason. For a more body-flattering setup, rest the mirror on the floor and lean it against a wall, tilted away from you. The angle will make you look taller and thinner.

But that doesn't mean you can't get culinary satisfaction along with the fat-busting, metabolism-enhancing benefits of smart, healthy nutrition. The exclusive Look Better Naked eating plan, designed by *Women's Health* advisor Keri Glassman, MS, RD, begins with a 2-day clean-food jump start that will push your body's reset button. In a single weekend, you'll shift your body and your mindset into optimal weight-loss mode, and then embark on an eating strategy that will help you lose up to 8 pounds in a month!

You'll Savor Delicious Food!

What do olive oil, nuts, and chocolate have in common? They're all yummy, but they're also packed with monounsaturated fats. Researchers studying the benefits of the Mediterranean diet, which abounds with these ingredients, discovered monounsaturated fats melt visceral belly fat as effectively as butter can be nuked in the microwave. You'll find them among the 20 Look Better Naked powerfoods, which also include lean meats, whole-grains, fruits and vegetables, and tasty treats such as cheese and peanut butter, and you'll eat them at every meal. The more you eat them, the more it will become second nature to include them in your diet. Instead of being one of those food-deprived, "restrained" eaters, you'll transform yourself into a "trained" eater—someone who is capable of eating what she wants, when she wants, and staying lean for life!

You'll Torch Fat and Build Tight, Toned Muscles!

There are plenty of ways to burn fat, and most of them take a very, very long time. Some involve running along the side of the road in pouring rain and sizzling heat. Some involve sweating away on a stairclimber in a stuffy gym, or slogging on a rowing machine on your lonely living room rug. And all of these methods have two things in common: They work slowly, and they're deadly boring. But there's a faster, easier way to burn more fat, in less time, and have more fun doing it. The exercise scientists who consult with *Women's Health* have studied every method of weight loss under the sun, and they've discovered an amazing fact: You need more iron. Not in your diet—in your hands.

According to the National Center for Health Statistics, a mere 21 percent of women do strength training two or more times a week. Yet when

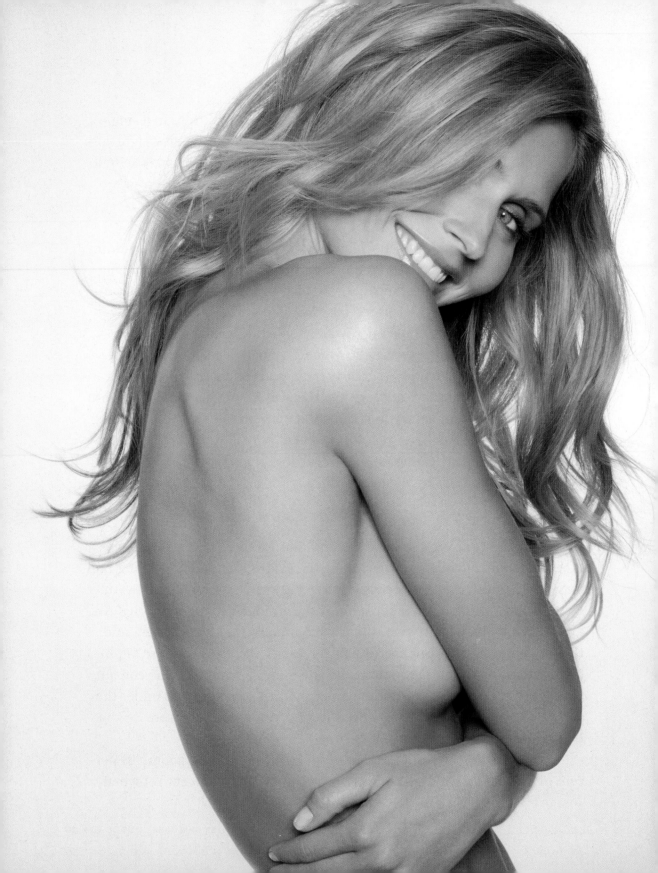

You need more iron! Not just in your diet but in your fitness routine, too.

you skip the weight room, you lose out on the ultimate flab melter. If you're one of the millions of women who have shied away from lifting weights for fear of bulking up, or because you're clueless about the right way to train, you're bound to become an iron-pumping convert once I show you an easy and ultraeffective way to achieve a hot body. It's called featherweight strength training. The twice-a-week workouts, designed by *Women's Health* contributor Rachel Cosgrove, a certified strength and conditioning specialist, will dramatically reduce overall body fat even without cutting a single calorie from your diet. Imagine trimming as many as 3 inches from your waist and hips and dropping an entire size (or two)! And all that new muscle will pay off in a long-term boost to your metabolism because your body will spend the 48 hours after a workout burning calories in order to help your muscles recover. That means you'll burn more calories, and more fat, all day, every day, even while you're relaxing in front of the TV. Good deal, right?

You'll Stand Taller—And Prouder!

One of the fastest, easiest ways to look and, especially, feel better is to change your posture. And no, that doesn't mean walking around with a dictionary balanced on your head. The Look Better Naked plan will literally lengthen your neck and spine, so that you stand—and sit—taller, and carry yourself with more authority.

Sitting at a desk for hours at a time destroys good posture and can result in a dysfunction that physical therapists call upper-cross syndrome. You probably know it as rounded shoulders. Even worse, research shows

You're not a slouch, but you may look like one. How important is standing up straight and dropping your shoulders? Correcting poor posture can make you look 5 pounds slimmer instantly!

that poor posture puts our abdominal muscles to sleep instead of challenging them to hold our bodies upright, further feeding our constant belly-bulging slump. (It's a particularly pesky problem for women who've had children, as stretched ab muscles and carrying kids can make it difficult for a woman to regain her full upright posture after delivery.) The good news: According to new research in the *European Journal of Social Psychology*, standing and sitting up straight is linked with higher levels of self-confidence. "Correcting poor posture can make you look 5 pounds slimmer instantly," says Deborah L. Mullen, a certified strength and conditioning specialist in San Luis Obispo, California. To keep that trim profile 24/7, you need to retrain and strengthen those belly-slimming, stand-tall muscles. We'll tell you how on starting in Chapter 4, but in the meantime stick a note to your computer that reads: SIT UP STRAIGHT, AND DROP YOUR SHOULDERS!

You'll Fine-Tune Your Hair, Skin, and Nails!

There's more to a naked-ready body than muscles and curves. Achieving smooth skin, a clear complexion, and strong hair and nails are part of the Look Better Naked program. That's because it's not just about how you look, but about how you feel—and details like these can have a major impact on your self-esteem. Take acne, for example: Studies have found that it can not only zap your desire to work out, but also that the presence of pimples can take a serious toll on self-perception—one that lingers long after you've graduated from high school! According to one report, people with acne often have greater levels of anxiety and depression than those with more serious chronic medical conditions. I don't mean to blow the importance of banishing acne or keeping your bikini line trimmed out of proportion, but I do want to underscore that Look Better Naked success, ultimately, is in the details—right down to the little parts of our bodies we fret over!

You'll Live a Longer, Healthier, Happier Life!

By choosing to eat better and live better, you'll lower your risk of developing a number of serious health problems. You already know most of this, but let's review: Excess fat is related to all sorts of illnesses, including chronic conditions such as heart disease, hypertension, and diabetes. Lose it and you'll be healthier! Excess belly fat is particularly problematic. Studies show that women whose waists measure 35 inches or more are at greater risk for heart disease and diabetes than women who are smaller around the middle. Trim it and you'll be healthier! Muscle mass does a body good in myriad ways: It supports the skeleton, revs metabolism (which helps to torch fat), and makes lifting everyday things easier (and safer!). Build it, and you'll be healthier! If you want to look—and feel— young and sexy and protect yourself from some of the most devastating diseases afflicting Americans today, you're holding the right tool.

That's a lot to promise for one book, and that's why you'll find every page packed with useful, practical, positive information that will begin making an impact on your life today.

Now let's get started!

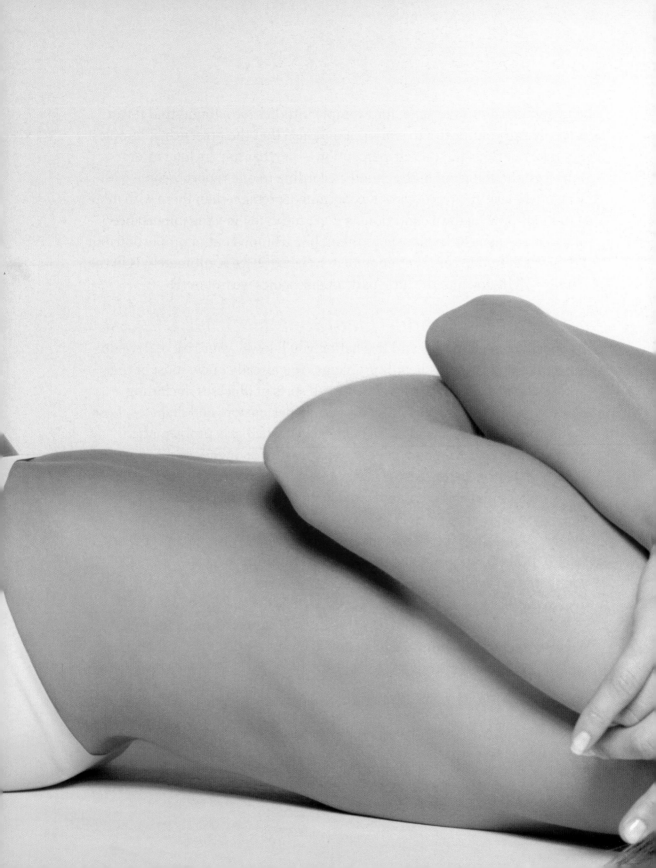

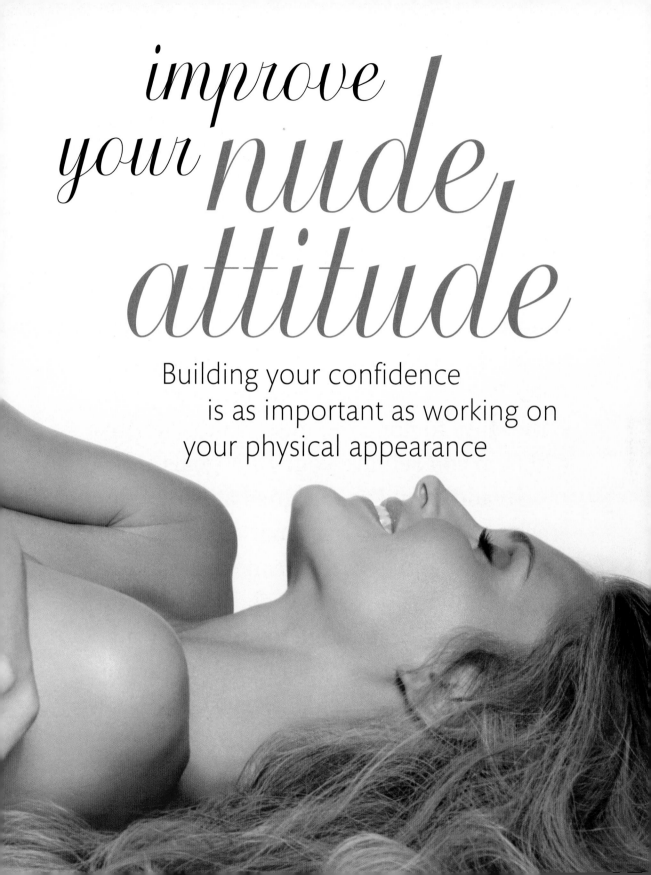

improve your nude attitude

Building your confidence
is as important as working on
your physical appearance

To *truly* look your best sans clothing, your brain needs to be as buff as your biceps. Allow me to explain: A strong, positive body image is as essential to reaching naked nirvana as streamlined thighs, a flat belly, or a smooth, dimple-free derriere. In this chapter, I'll spell out why training your brain to embrace your body is a critical part of the *Look Better Naked* program, and give you some ways to hone the mental muscles that will help you achieve your *LBN* goals.

In addition, I've designed a 6-week-long crash course of body-sensual activities on page 28, to jump-start this mental make-over. You'll do one each week, after which time you'll be better able to appreciate all the awesome things your body does for you, and, in turn, begin to like the way it looks a lot more. First, though, let's go over why that's so important.

What Is *Body Image*, Anyway?

You might think body image is simply the mental picture you have of your physical self. And you would be right—to an extent. But what you see with your mind's eye isn't the whole story. Most experts also include in the definition of body image how a person experiences her body, the *emotions* that arise when she considers her physique. It's pretty straightforward, really: If, when you encounter a mirror, you can think things like "I'm pretty" or "I'm strong" or "I look damn hot in this bikini (or out of it!)," then you've got a healthy, positive body image. But if there's a nagging little voice in your head constantly throwing confidence-crushing curveballs at you—like "my butt is too big" or "my breasts are too small"—then your body image might need a little work. And it matters not (or, at least, not much) what the reality of your physical appearance is. Says Amy L. Flowers, PhD, a psychologist in Macon, Georgia: "In my body image workshops, I've seen overweight women who truly like how they look, and slender ones who hate their appearance."

Chances are, you have a pretty good idea of how you feel about your body—i.e., whether the overall image you have of yourself is positive, negative, or somewhere in between. And that is vitally important to how you look to others. When people feel good about their bodies, they come across as more attractive, says Flowers. Adds Rita Freedman, PhD, who also specializes in self-image issues: "People pick up on the vibes that you send out about your self feelings." Think about

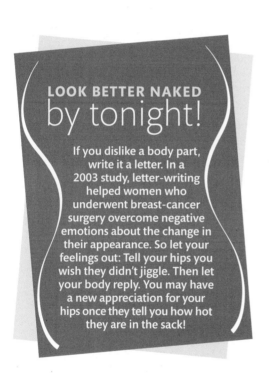

LOOK BETTER NAKED
by tonight!

If you dislike a body part, write it a letter. In a 2003 study, letter-writing helped women who underwent breast-cancer surgery overcome negative emotions about the change in their appearance. So let your feelings out: Tell your hips you wish they didn't jiggle. Then let your body reply. You may have a new appreciation for your hips once they tell you how hot they are in the sack!

it: If you're so self-conscious in the presence of others, even a significant other, that you spend all your time trying to keep what you perceive to be your "big butt" facing the wall or your "small breasts" hidden from view, you'll hardly wow your audience. In fact, if that audience happens to be male, negativity can make or break his attraction to you, according to a study in *Archives of Sexual Behavior*. When a group of 50 men were

Do You Dislike Your Body *Too* Much?

help
If these sound familiar, find a therapist near you by searching for "BDD Referral Listings" at butler.org.

It's one thing to think you might look better minus a few pounds. It's an altogether different thing to be obsessed with what you perceive as your physical flaws. In that case, you might suffer from body dysmorphic disorder, or BDD—what's sometimes even referred to as the "disorder of imagined ugliness."

According to the Anxiety Disorders Association of America, BDD is a condition in which a person is persistently preoccupied with an imagined or slight physical defect. This perception of imperfection could be focused on any part of the body, and may be so pervasive that a person with BDD spends hours obsessing about it. She may think she looks ugly, abnormal, even deformed.

That said, the ADAA estimates that only about 1 percent of the population has BDD. Think you might be in that minority?

Here are some signs of BDD:
• *Going to lengths to cover up the "flaw" (with clothing, makeup, even the way you position your body)*
• *Comparing your body part of concern with that of others*
• *Considering surgery*
• *Constantly checking yourself in a mirror or avoiding mirrors altogether*
• *Picking at your skin*
• *Grooming excessively*
• *Working out incessantly*
• *Repeatedly changing your clothes*

asked to discuss what they found arousing—or not—several volunteered that a woman's self-esteem could affect their libido. Said one, "If you were with a girl that just hates her body and just doesn't want you to see it, that is a total turnoff."

It's not hard to see why bolstering your mental attitude toward your physical appearance is doubly important when it comes to baring all, because when you're nude, there's nothing to camouflage (or smooth or lift) the parts you're dissatisfied with. But in some ways, training your brain to think happier thoughts about your body is the easiest part of the LBN plan, because with a little effort, achieving a healthy self-image is possible for everyone. And once you learn how to muzzle the negatives that mess with your head when you think about your bare body, you'll come across as sexier and more confident—whether you're dressed or nude—and you'll experience that change before you drop an ounce, pick up a dumbbell, or wax a spare hair. Step one: Understanding why we're so squeamish about letting it all hang out in the first place.

The Not-So-Naked Apes

We humans are the only members of the animal kingdom who keep our bodies covered under most circumstances. *Homo sapiens* probably began wearing clothes (well, in those pre-PETA days, animal skins) around the time they figured out the magic that happens when you rub two sticks together. "Once people harnessed fire, about one and a half million years ago, they could move to colder climates in order to hunt," says Helen Fisher, PhD, a biological anthropologist at Rutgers University, "so clothing has probably been around at least since then."

But the theory that humans started wrapping up to stay toasty on the tundra doesn't explain why people in all climates, even the hottest ones, cover up to some degree. There are very few cultures in which people don't at least wear some version of a loincloth, says Fisher. Much of the reason for that has to do with the comfort and protection of the private parts. (Would you want to plop *your* bare behind down on the hot sand of the

Sahara or a brambly forest floor?) But it's also grounded in mankind's modesty about genitals—which, when you think about it, seems almost absurd, given that we all start out buck-naked.

One explanation for the genesis of that modesty is, of course, the biblical one. According to the story of Adam and Eve, the very first insight those two gleaned upon biting into the forbidden fruit of the Tree of Knowledge was that they were naked—and, more to the point, that there was something *wrong* with that. They each grabbed the nearest, biggest fig leaf they could find and covered what they suddenly perceived as their "private" parts. It's hard to tell in illustrations how the first couple got their vegetative Skivvies to stay in place—yet another miracle, perhaps—but the point is, they were intuitively ashamed of their nakedness.

The tale of Adam and Eve certainly helps to explain how the collective consciousness of most Western cultures became enmeshed in the idea, that in order to be acceptable, you have to keep certain body parts under wraps. But according to Fisher, there's also a biological explanation for why we began covering up. "Sexual behavior is an important aspect of who we are; it leads to reproduction, which leads to the continuation of the human race," she explains. "For that reason, every culture in the world has codes for controlling sexuality within their communities, especially in terms of who mates with whom, and under what circumstances—we copulate in private, for example. Having social mores that require us to keep our sexual organs out of sight enables us to

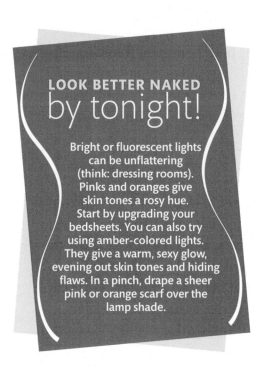

LOOK BETTER NAKED
by tonight!

Bright or fluorescent lights can be unflattering (think: dressing rooms). Pinks and oranges give skin tones a rosy hue. Start by upgrading your bedsheets. You can also try using amber-colored lights. They give a warm, sexy glow, evening out skin tones and hiding flaws. In a pinch, drape a sheer pink or orange scarf over the lamp shade.

walk around without sending sexual signals to each other in public. It's how we control who we turn on." In other words, it's a way to guarantee that we don't turn on the wrong person.

That may make sense, but what doesn't is why being nude in *private* is so uncomfortable for many people—especially women. (Most guys seem happy to strip down under pretty much any condition; more on that later.) Here's where the importance of body image comes in. When I asked the 3,500 *Women's Health* readers in my Look Better Naked survey, "Do you think you look better naked or clothed?" nearly three-quarters went with "clothed." What's more, a mere 8 percent said they were proud of their bare bodies. The implication is that many of us females don't like to wear our birthday suits because we don't like how they're cut, or how they fit, or the way they're trimmed. The problem is, our dissatisfaction always seems to stem from what's currently "in fashion" for the female physique. Which turns out to be anything but a steady target. As a 2002 study in the *Journal of Sexual Research* found, the waist-to-hip ratio (WHR) for *Playboy* centerfolds and Miss America winners has changed dramatically through the decades—yet not as you might expect. The "preferred value," the authors concluded, "decreased in the early through mid-20th century and then increased in the mid- to late-20th century."

How to Boost Your Body Image

It's one thing to understand why you may not be frolicking around nude all the time. It's quite another to do something about it. That's where the Look Better Naked plan comes in. The diet, workout, and grooming tips in the chapters that follow are guaranteed to get you to your personal best physically (emphasis on *your* personal best). But getting there won't matter one iota if you don't develop the mindset to go along with the physical improvements you make. "You can 'fix' your 'flaws,'" says Freedman, "but if *you* still see them, you're never going to portray yourself as a confident person." Angel Williams, a fitness trainer and performer in Montclair, New Jersey, seconds that emotion: "People see what you offer.

If your vibe is, 'I feel beautiful,' then people will see you that way." Obtaining a "beautiful vibe" might take some work, but it's worth it.

Fake it till you make it. When it comes to the image you project to others, "the way you use your body is far more important than what it looks like," says Paul Dobransky, MD, a psychiatrist and the founder of womenshappiness.com, a Web site devoted to relationships. The key is to project confidence. If you stand taller, pull your shoulders back, and stride across the room with purpose, you're guaranteed no one will be thinking, "Wow, she sure could stand to lose a few."

Pay a compliment forward. Women can be highly competitive about their bodies: Deep down, we are, after all, flaunting our potential in order to nab a guy and keep the human race ticking along. ("May the wispiest waist win!") You could argue, then, that it's our role in the survival of the species to compare, contrast, and criticize—and as a result we're sometimes less than free with the flattery. So when a woman compliments another woman, the words can carry considerably more weight than when a man does.

The point is, the more positive feedback you get from other females about your appearance, the more positive your body image will be. The best way to invite compliments? Offer them up yourself. No need to be disingenuous; I'm not suggesting you start passing out plaudits like Halloween candy. But go ahead and tell the woman ahead of you in line at Starbucks that you love her haircut. You'll feel good for making someone else feel good—and you'll create the kind of karma that will bring self-esteem-enhancing kudos your way.

Say "om." Yoga can work wonders for improving body image. A 2005 study published in the *Psychology of Women Quarterly*, for example, found that women who did yoga were less likely to objectify their bodies and were more satisfied with their appearance than those who did only aerobics or who did no exercise at all. In addition, the women who did other forms of exercise (specifically, running and aerobics) were more likely to have the types of negative feelings about their bodies that are associated with conditions such as anorexia or bulimia.

Why does yoga have such a body-affirming effect? "Yoga means to 'yoke together,' referring to mind, body, and spirit," explains Jan St. John, who's been a yoga instructor for more than 20 years. "Other fitness classes are externally directed, while a yoga class should be internally directed, with the teacher as guide, rather than someone who's placing demands on her students. It's an hour that belongs to you, and should be an opportunity not to judge your body, but to appreciate it."

The key to improving body image through yoga is to choose the right kind. St. John recommends Iyengar, which flows from posture to posture at a relatively slow pace. You can try that one, or any other that's ever intersted you!

Dance, dance, dance. A dance class (or dance-inspired workout) can loosen you up and make you feel sexy, something that functional training—Spinning, say, or running—can't do. "Dancing is a liberator of all the things that hold us back," says Williams—and that includes negative feelings we have about our bodies. In a dance class, you have to face the mirror. Look for a class that allows you to move your body freely, such as hip-hop, belly dancing, jazz, and many types of dance with Latin or African roots. The key is to give it time: "You're not going to connect on day one," says Williams. "You have to show up regularly and challenge yourself. If you commit to that, you'll begin to notice little things about your body, how it's changing and what it can do. You'll start to appreciate it more and more. Eventually you'll be saying to yourself, 'Wow, my body was able to do this,' and you'll look at yourself differently." Even when you're naked.

21%
of women say that they never have sex with the lights on!

6
ways to
feel
Sexier

▶ In order to feel more self-assured, attractive, and sexy in your own (bare) skin, you're going to need to spend time doing things unclothed besides just showering and having sex. I'm not suggesting anything extreme—just an assortment of activities to do over the course of the program, designed to gently nudge you out of your covered-up comfort zone. You'll do one activity per week, but feel free to repeat any or all that you find especially confidence-boosting!

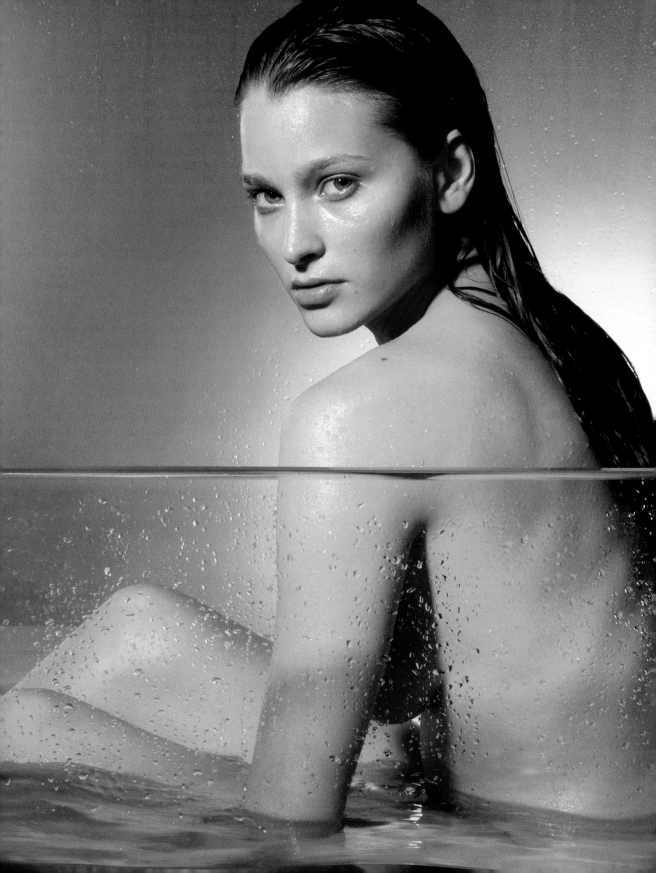

take a bath

➡ If you're like most people, you don't spend much more than 8 to 10 minutes in the shower. Bathing in the tub will help you to slow down your ablutions and will give you the perfect opportunity to become better acquainted with your body all over again.

Max Out The Experience:

• **Schedule your bath for when you'll really have the time to devote to it.** Don't cheat and try to fit it in before work. Rushing through the process will defeat the point. Make sure you won't be interrupted, either: Leave your cell phone in another room and lock the door if you don't live alone.

• **Make yourself feel great.** Use a scented bath oil, pour a glass of wine (you might want to use a plastic cup), pipe in some soft music. If it's nighttime, light candles in lieu of flipping on the overhead; for that matter, close the shades and burn candles even if it's daytime. Setting the stage this way might sound corny, but the point is to indulge and pamper *all* your senses. "If the goal is to get comfy nude, the more reinforcements you can put around yourself, the better," says Barbara Keesling, PhD, a sex therapist and author of *How To Make Love All Night*.

• **Don't lather up right away.** Instead, just relax. Pay attention to how the water feels on your body. Create gentle waves and notice how it feels as the water moves over your skin.

• **Use a soft cloth to wash up.** This is no time to scrub yourself silly with a loofah. Start with your feet and touch every part of your body from your soles on up. Take it slow! Appreciate how good the cloth feels against your skin, and how pleasant it is to focus on yourself.

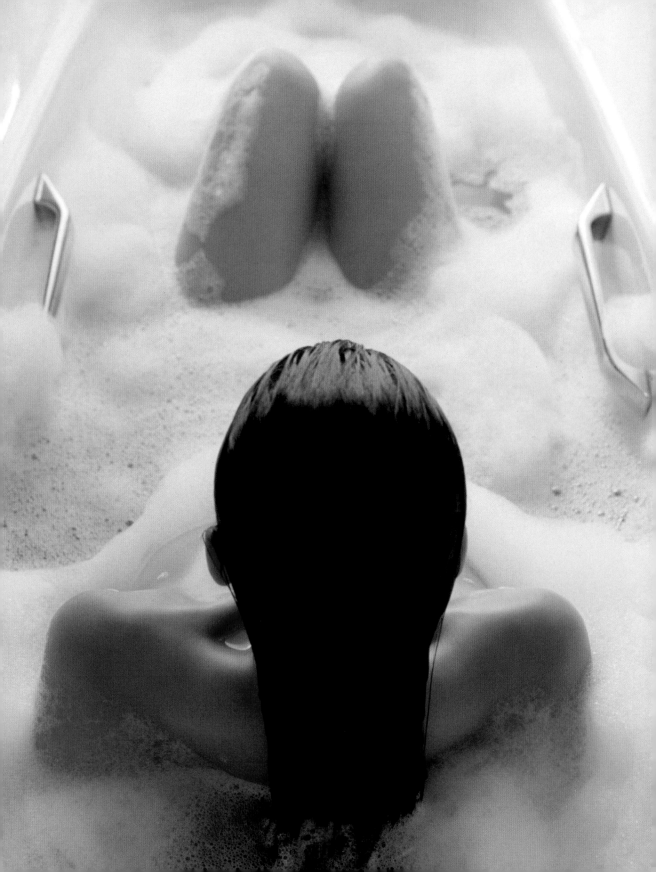

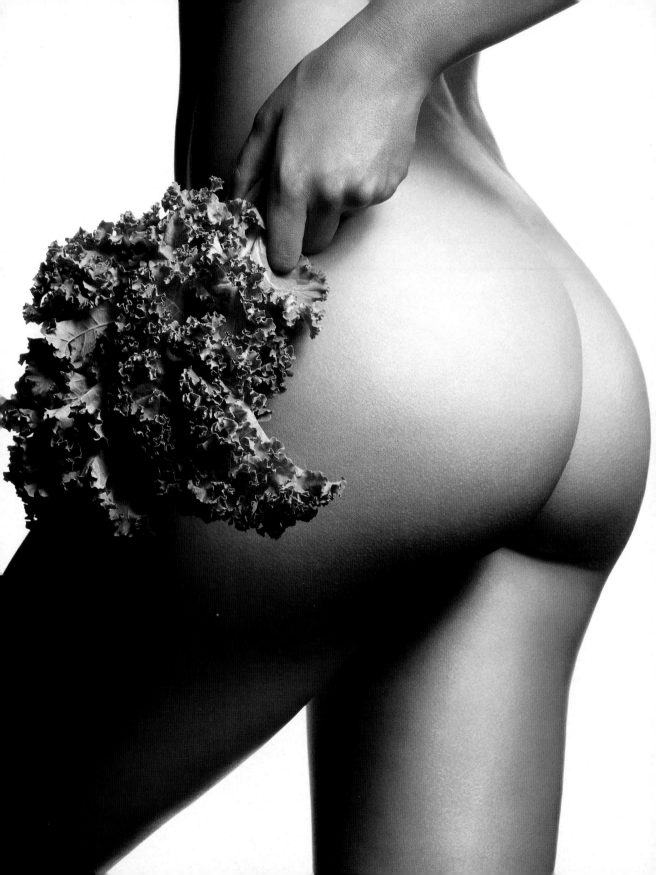

share dinner in the *nude*

▶▶ Next to sex, eating is the most sensual thing we do. It engages every sense—even hearing, as we crunch into a crisp apple, say, or sip a spoonful of soup. A romantic dinner is often the prelude to lovemaking. (Or even a part of it, for some couples!) It sustains us and is vital to our very well-being. And yet, we almost always do it clothed—for obvious reasons, of course. But, for the purposes of becoming more comfortable in the nude, there's much to be said for pairing nakedness with a delicious meal, says Keesling. "We used to do it all the time in sex therapy school!" she admits.

Max Out The Experience:

• **Serve finger foods.** You'll feel considerably less awkward eating cheese and crackers with your hands than you would juggling utensils or sawing through a lamb chop with a steak knife while naked.

• **Make the meal pretty.** Simple fare is fine, but you want it to be pleasing to look at. Don't just slap those crackers on a paper plate—arrange them on a platter, with a selection of luscious fruit, perhaps. An assortment of sushi can make for an ideal nude meal: It's colorful and filling.

• **Dine picnic style.** Spread out a big, soft, stain-resistant (you don't want to have to be fussy about spills) blanket on the floor and enjoy your feast there. Keep the lighting low; you'll feel less self-conscious. Candlelight or the light from a fire will cast flattering shadows on your skin.

• **Eat mindfully.** "Take your time; eat in slow motion," says Lori Buckley, PhD, of the Center for Relationship, Marriage, and Sex Therapy in Pasadena, California. "Look at the food, smell it; be aware of the way it feels in your mouth, and the flavors it leaves behind." Make every bite a sensuous experience.

Snooze
in the nude

▶▶ More than half of the women who responded to my Look Better Naked survey reported that they never sleep naked. But for the purposes of getting used to spending time au naturel, leaving your pj's in the drawer for a night is a worthy experience. You'll be in your own home and no one will see you (except your partner, if you have one, and he won't mind a bit—trust me). But to get the most out of your naked 8 hours, don't just climb into bed, strip under the covers, and go straight to sleep. Spend some time experiencing the sensation of being sans nightie before you doze off. If you like the way your sheets make you feel, splurge on a new set that has a higher thread count than you're used to and make it a regular thing.

Max Out
The Experience:

• **Start slow.** If it's warm enough in your bedroom, lie on your back on top of the covers, close your eyes, and relax your muscles one by one, starting with your toes and moving up your body to your shoulders, neck, and even facial muscles. If by any chance there's a breeze in your room, from an open window or ceiling fan, say, tune in to the feeling of the air as it moves across your bare skin.

• **Focus on your skin.** After you slip between the sheets, pay attention to how the fabric feels on different areas of your body— particularly the ones that are usually buffered from them by nightclothes.

• **Get comfy.** Try lying in different positions, both to find the one that's most comfortable for snoozing, and to vary the sensations you experience.

• **Hit "snooze."** When you wake up in the morning, don't get up right away; spend a little time luxuriating in the comfort of your bed. Stretch your arms above your head, reach your toes toward the footboard, do whatever feels good to unkink your body before you get up. And when you do: bonus points for heading to the bathroom minus your robe!

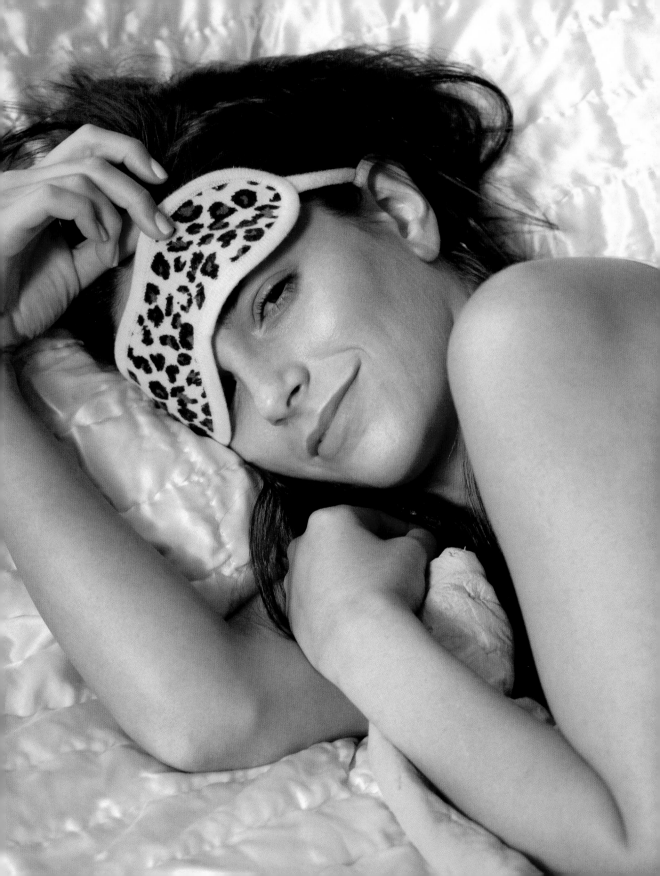

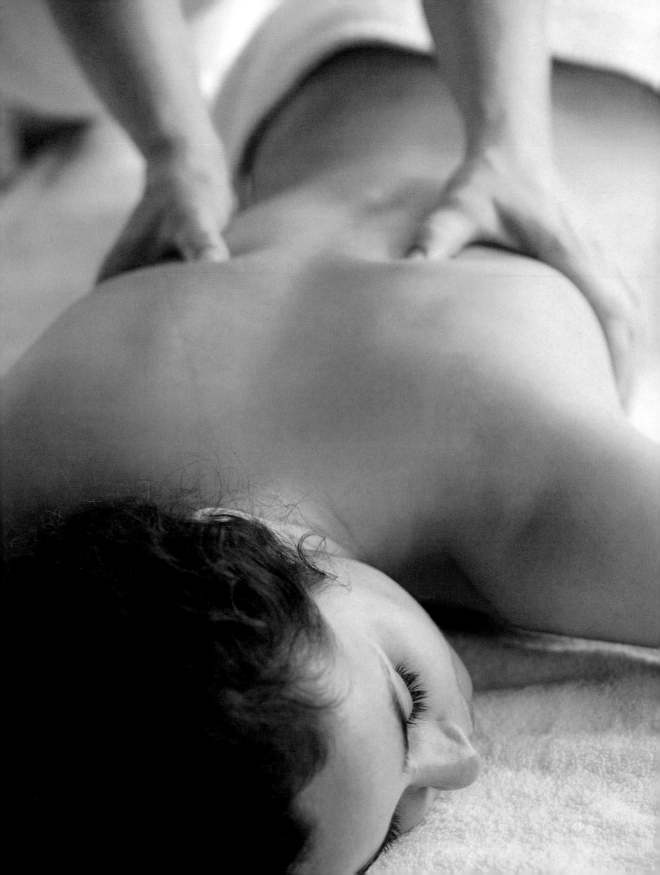

get a Massage

This step is a way to "practice" being nude by spending time in an environment where it's okay. It's also an effective way of becoming more closely acquainted with your body, so that you can grow to like and appreciate it more. How you approach this particular "exercise," and what you glean from it, however, will depend in part on how much massage experience you already have. If you've never had a professional massage (and especially if the reason for that is because you feel uncomfortable having a stranger see and touch your body), getting one may feel like jumping into the deep end. But that, of course, is the point: I want you to go ahead and get naked, and I promise that this will be one of the most enjoyable ways to do that. The most important thing to remember if you're squeamish is this: The therapist will not be judging you in any way. "I've had people apologize for not shaving their legs," says MK Brennan, past president of the American Massage Therapy Association. "Believe me, the massage therapist will be focused only on what's going on underneath your skin: the musculature and any tense areas that might need extra attention."

Max Out The Experience:

• **Book a Swedish massage.** What you're looking for is a light, gentle, full-body experience that consists of flowing, nonstop strokes, designed to relax and rejuvenate you—not a heavy-hitting, deep-tissue Shiatsu treatment.

• **Be up-front with the practitioner.** Tell her (or him—make the request when you make your appointment) about any qualms you're having, especially in regard to undressing. She'll explain that you'll be draped with sheets that she'll move around as she works and only the part of your body that's being tended to will be uncovered. Your breasts and pelvis will never be exposed, assures Brennan.

• **Pay attention.** Notice how it feels as the massage therapist adjusts her strokes. Be aware when she stops to work on a specific area: It means that she's feeling tension in the muscles there, which is a clue to where your body takes on stress. Ask her to explain what she's doing as she goes along—especially if you think you're likely to doze off! That will also help to strengthen the mind-body connection that a massage encourages.

• **Make an evening of it.** In a pinch, your partner can do the honors. Have him stick to long, gentle strokes—no tickling or kneeding—and use an oil-based lubricant or a lotion. (If he uses too much, his hands will slip off your skin rather than glide over it.) Above all, enjoy!

get fitted for Sexy lingerie

▶ Like a massage therapist, a professional lingerie fitter will take an objective view of your body. Unlike a massage therapist, she'll go over with you what she sees as she measures you and evaluates the items you try on. Pay attention to what she says: She sees dozens of nearly nude bodies every day, and her reactions to yours will underscore just how normal it is—and, more important, what your best assets are.

Max Out The Experience:

• **Go to a boutique** (or the lingerie section of a high-end department store). Sure, you can pick up a three-for-$25 array of panties at a big chain store. You can even get a salesgirl to help you out. But I guarantee that she won't be a pro who's been trained to fit bras and other underthings correctly.

• **Be clear about what you're looking for.** Don't be coy. "Tell the salesperson that you're self-conscious about your rear end, for example, or that you especially hate your love handles," says Dee Generallo, who's been fitting bras and swimwear for more than 6 years at a New York-area lingerie boutique. Number one, she won't bat an eye. Number two, she may well point out that what you think you see in the mirror is not at all what she's seeing straight on. Not that she'll lie, but she'll be much kinder about your "flaws" than you are. Try picking up the language she uses and applying it to yourself after you leave the store.

• **Let her see you.** Don't just try things on and then snatch them off before the fitter has a chance to weigh in. Even if you're sure an item is all wrong for you, by actually seeing how it fits she can figure out what might work better.

• **Buy something.** If you can't afford the $200 bit o' lace that so prettily enhances your breasts, opt for a less extravagant purchase. A thong is a good choice, especially if you've never worn one. Having a little secret underneath your street clothes can help you feel sexy and confident. At the very least, take home this lesson about your body: While it may not be perfect, while you may have areas you'd like to change, it's yours, and it's beautiful in its own right.

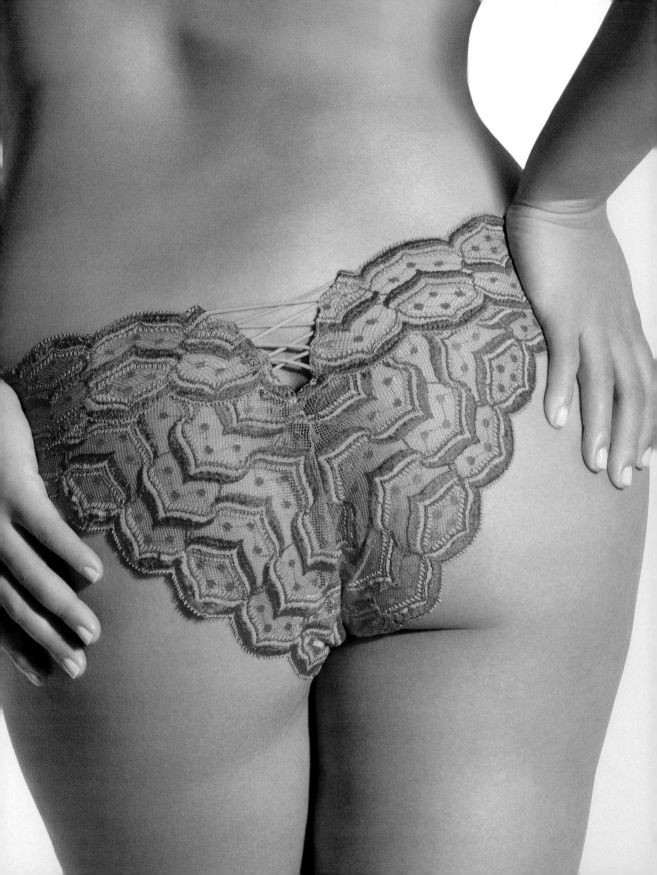

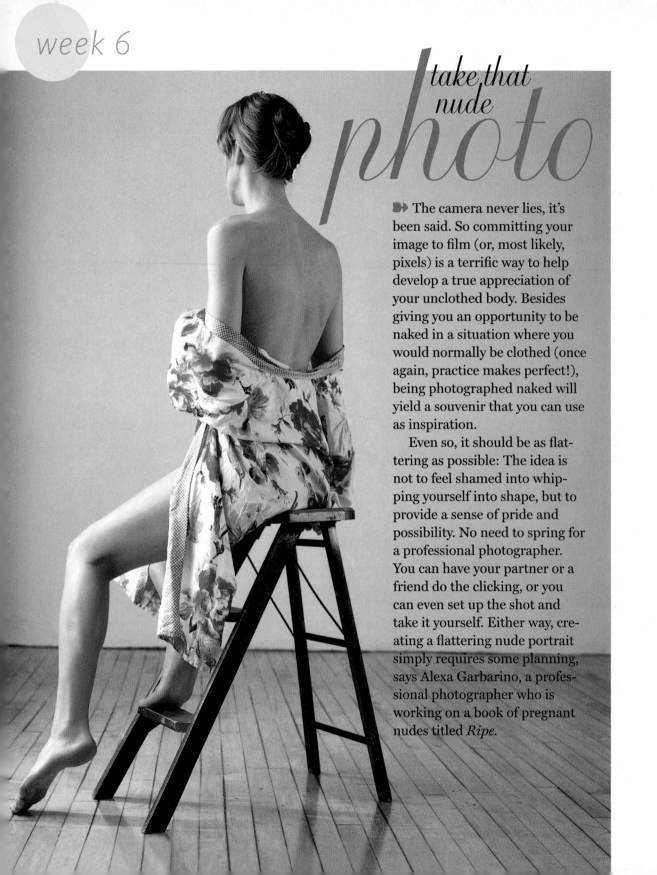

take that nude *photo*

➡ The camera never lies, it's been said. So committing your image to film (or, most likely, pixels) is a terrific way to help develop a true appreciation of your unclothed body. Besides giving you an opportunity to be naked in a situation where you would normally be clothed (once again, practice makes perfect!), being photographed naked will yield a souvenir that you can use as inspiration.

Even so, it should be as flattering as possible: The idea is not to feel shamed into whipping yourself into shape, but to provide a sense of pride and possibility. No need to spring for a professional photographer. You can have your partner or a friend do the clicking, or you can even set up the shot and take it yourself. Either way, creating a flattering nude portrait simply requires some planning, says Alexa Garbarino, a professional photographer who is working on a book of pregnant nudes titled *Ripe.*

*Max Out
The Experience:*

- **Build your courage.** Look at the works of some masters of nude photography such as Ruth Bernhard, Helmut Newton, Edward Weston, and Jock Sturges. Not only will you become more comfortable with viewing the naked body in all its glory, you'll see just how diverse the human form is (in other words, you'll come to realize that every body is beautiful in its own way). Notice how the photographers use light to cast shadows on some body parts and illuminate others, and pay attention to how the models are posed. It'll help you figure out how you want to set up your own shot.

- **Stick to black and white.** It's less distracting than color, and you'll see fewer irregularities in skin tone.

- **Light it right.** Soft, diffused light will soften any lumps, bumps, or other imperfections on your skin. If you have the privacy to pose outdoors, a photograph taken on a cloudy day or in the early morning just as the sun is rising will yield the most flattering effects. If you'll be shooting indoors, close the curtains if the sun is streaming in, or put a gauzy curtain over a lamp.

- **Get comfy.** Choose a spot where you feel both physically and psychologically at ease. If you're anxious or uncomfortable, it'll show in your photo. Put on some relaxing music and have a glass of wine to help you loosen up.

- **Create a "clean line" as you pose.** If you're standing, keep your legs together, with one foot slightly in front of the other. This way there'll be no "negative space" between your legs; when they're slightly overlapped, they'll look thinner too. If you're reclining, stretch out and raise your arms above your head: This will diminish natural body folds.

- **Mind your breasts:** They can be tricky, especially if you're well endowed. Gravity is going to make them look saggy (which will in turn create an unattractive shadow beneath them). Try reclining on a sofa or sitting back on a chair, with your arms raised above your head, to lift them.

- **Focus on the contours.** This photograph isn't about honing in on specific details; it's about capturing your unique shape, in all its beauty and possibility. So if you don't want your breasts or nether regions to show, go ahead and cover them up. For example, lie on your side and drape one leg over the other; cross your hands across your chest à la pregnant Demi Moore on that famous cover of *Vanity Fair*. Or simply have the photograph taken from behind; you won't feel as exposed but you'll get the experience of being photographed au naturel.

Why guys don't mind

BARING THEIR BUTTS

(not to mention everything else)

➠ In case you haven't noticed, most males won't hesitate to strip down. They'll do it to cool off, to get more comfortable, to take a spontaneous dip— and, of course, they'll get naked in a heartbeat if there's the smallest chance that doing so will lead to having sex. Even if a man grabs a towel when caught in the buff, it's highly unlikely that he's covering up because he happens to be embarrassed by his body—no matter what kind of shape he's in. A beer belly, a pimply bum, a rug of back hair, even a member that's on the modest side is unlikely to prevent the average dude from flaunting it all. The reason a man attempts to keep things under wraps? It's what polite people are supposed to do.

Women, on the other hand, are much less willing to let it all hang out. My LBN survey found, for example, that 83 percent of the 3,500 women who responded take pains to cover themselves in the gym locker room; only a minority will peel off their sweaty workout clothes and saunter to the shower without trying to cover up at least some part of their anatomy with one of those postage-stamp-size bits of terry cloth that pass as towels at most health clubs. Half of the respondents grab a robe or T-shirt after rolling out of bed, and only a handful feel more comfortable being naked in front of a friend than in front of their husband or boyfriend.

So why are guys able to frolic in a naked comfort zone that's so much larger than most women's?

According to anthropologist Helen Fisher, it comes back to the innate desire of humans to procreate.

In their drive to keep the human race going, men are on the lookout for a partner who can produce healthy babies, and certain attributes of the female body are excellent indicators of that. The most important of these is the size of a woman's waist in relation to her hips—what's technically known as waist-hip ratio, or WHR. "Women whose waist measurements are 70 percent of their hip

Our ideals of beauty are driven by our desire to keep the human race alive. So when men and women undress, a woman is advertising a good deal more than a man is.

measurements are most likely to get pregnant and bear healthy young," says Fisher. Calculate your own waist-hip ratio by dividing the circumference of your waist by the circumference of your hips at their widest part. The "ideal" result would be 0.7 or thereabouts. So, for example, if your waist measures 25 inches and your hips measure 34 inches, your WHR would be 0.735—just about "perfect."

Studies have found that women with a waist-hip ratio of around 0.7 have optimal levels of estrogen and tend to be less susceptible to heart disease, diabetes, and ovarian cancer. There's even evidence that babies born to women with wide hips and a low WHR are more intelligent. All of this means that, ultimately, men are most

attracted to women who'll make them proud papas of smart, healthy children—women whose middles curve inward in the classic hourglass shape. It's the reason for the corsets and bustles of the past, and the crunches and Pilates of the present. At the very core of what makes us human, our ideals of what's beautiful are driven by our unshakable need to keep the human race alive.

More to the point, it means that "when men and women undress, a woman is advertising a great deal more than a man is," adds Fisher. This leaves males freer to flaunt their foibles, because women are programmed to judge a potential mate by nonphysical attributes— his ability to protect and care for a future family financially, for example.

what to Eat

to look better naked!

A healthfully hedonistic diet
that will cleanse your body,
help you lose unwanted pounds,
and teach you to eat right for life

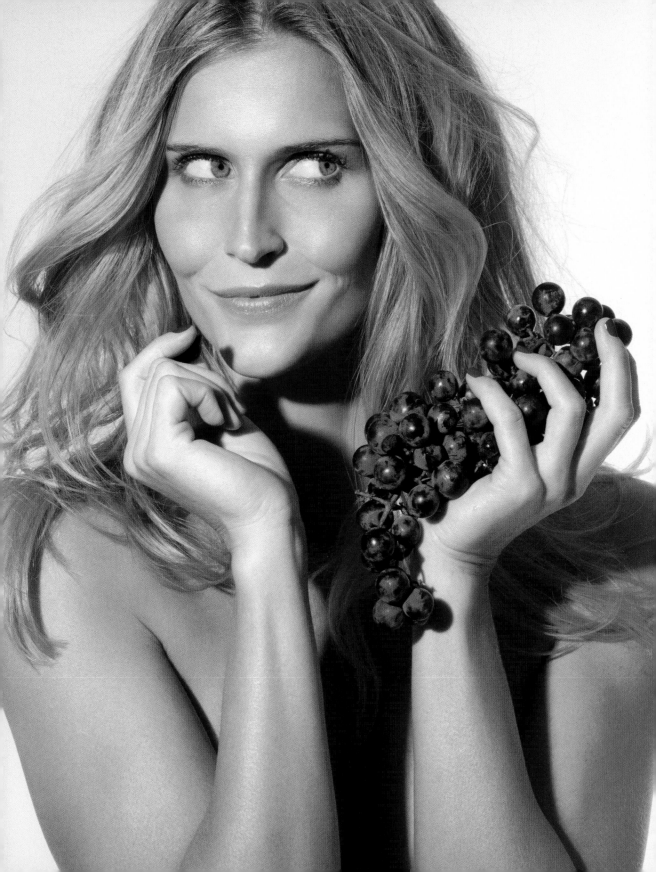

I know what you're thinking: YUCK, A DIET. The d-word word has rather evil connotations—hunger, deprivation, and drudgery, to name just a few. Then there are also the major inconveniences of not *really* being able to eat at restaurants or meet friends for after-work drinks. Evil, indeed. Fortunately, the Look Better Naked eating plan requires none of those things. The only catch: You'll have to hit the supermarket and spend a little time in the kitchen, but probably no more than you would have otherwise.

The following plan isn't merely a weight-loss program designed to help you peel off any extra pounds that are standing between the now-you and the new-you (though it will absolutely accomplish that). No, this plan will do much, much more by changing how you even *think* about food. It's the brainchild of *Women's Health* nutrition advisor Keri Glassman, MS, RD. Glassman, who's my own nutrition guru, is all about treating the body to things that are good for it. She told me this once, and it's probably the best nutrition tip I've ever heard: Learn to focus on what you can eat—not what you can't or shouldn't. "The point is to empower yourself," says Glassman. "Train yourself to stop thinking, 'I *can't* have chocolate cake.' Think 'I can have delicious blueberries' instead. If you think can't, you'll feel miserable and deprived—or you'll go ahead and indulge anyway, and end up feeling even worse. By choosing to eat something as good for you as those sweet, luscious, nutrient-packed berries, you take control of what you put into your body, which will in turn help you to feel positive about yourself—*and* still lose weight."

To that end, the LBN diet is healthfully hedonistic. Because Glassman has incorporated all sorts of dietary luxuries, your tastebuds should do a little happy dance at every meal. You'll eat cheese, nuts, waffles, pork, avocado, and peanut butter—and you'll even have a go-to signature cocktail for when you're out with friends! During the course of the program, you won't do without, you'll do *with*—and you'll *enjoy* feeding your body, rather than resent all the trouble you have to go to in order to

LOOK BETTER NAKED
by tonight!

Research has found that calcium-rich foods can help deflate puffiness from six-pack saboteurs such as pre-period puffiness and the inflating effects of salty foods. It'll take about 1,000 milligrams of the bone-building stuff to win the battle of the temporary bulge—a cup of low-fat milk, 8 ounces of low-fat yogurt, and a 2½ ounce serving of low-fat cheese over the course of a day ought to do it.

slim it down. In fact, I'm hoping that you'll appreciate the food in this plan so much that you'll eat slowly and really savor it, because it turns out that your grandmother was onto something when she scolded you for not chewing your food. According to research in the *British Medical Journal,* you're 84 percent more likely to be overweight if you eat quickly. Meanwhile, across the English Channel, Dutch researchers have determiwned that people who chew food for 9 seconds eat much less than those who chew for an average of 3 seconds. And a recent study in the *Journal of Clinical Endocrinology & Metabolism* revealed one possible reason: Eating fast may stymie the release of hormones that help regulate appetite.

The majority of the ingredients in this diet are included not just for their weight-loss or palate-pampering properties. Look Better Naked foods have natural elements that will enhance your appearance—by targeting belly fat, plumping up skin cells, "glowifying" your complexion, adding luster to your hair, strengthening your nails, and even protecting you from illness. (Knowing that you're doing everything you can to dodge chronic problems such as cancer and heart disease should go a long way toward hiking your body confidence.) What's more, Glassman has perked up the plan with a wealth of flavor boosters—spice mixtures, salsas, sauces, and dips. Many of them are low-cal freebies that you can sprinkle/stir/rub into your food with abandon. Whether you choose to mix them into canned tuna, scramble them with eggs, or add them atop steamed vegetables, do so to your mouth's content. Experimenting with different flavors and textures can be fun, and will make eating that much more pleasurable. Plus, many of the ingredients in these flavor boosters qualify as LBN foods by containing feel-good/look-good properties. You'll learn

Diet designed by **Keri Glassman, MS, RD**, author of *The 02 Diet: The Cutting Edge Antioxidant-Based Program That Will Make You Healthy and Beautiful,* and president of Keri Glassman, Nutritious Life, a nutrition counseling practice (nutritiouslife.com).

more later about all the LBN foods and exactly what they can do for you, but hopefully you're no longer thinking YUCK. More like YUM, right? Well, there's even more to love:

You'll Never Count Calories!

Glassman's taken care of all the tabulating. Eat the portions as they're written and you'll be right on target—about 1,400 calories per day. Most women will lose 1 to 2 pounds a week at that level, as long as you're also following the fitness program in Chapter 4.

You'll Be Able to Splurge—At Least Occasionally!

All too often, one mistake can put you on a slippery slope, no matter how conscientious you are about following a prescribed diet. You'll indulge, say, in a slice of chocolate cake at a party, decide that this one infraction means you've failed altogether and you might as well give up—and then you'll, well, give up. The LBN plan gets around this all-or-nothing trap by allowing for two slipups every 21 days. In other words, while ideally you'll stick to the diet every day, if over the course of 3 weeks you find yourself straying off the plan, it's okay as long as it happens just once in a while. "If you do splurge on something, try to stop when you're satisfied, and round out the 'forbidden' food with plenty of healthy ones," says Glassman.

You Won't Spend Hours Cooking!

There are no elaborate recipes in this diet. If you're a kitchen-shy, takeout kind of person, there's not a single meal here that will intimidate you. These are the only four kitchen skills you'll need: baking, sautéing, scrambling, and grilling. If you know how to do those—and I'm not sure I can help you if you can't!—you'll be just fine. If you're ever short on time, you can also opt for precooked ingredients, such as grilled chicken or steamed veggies, as long as you make sure they don't have added fat and calories. And if you're a gourmet, just add the no-calorie flourishes to the ingredients in each meal—that's what the flavor boosters are for!

You'll Eat Healthier Foods!

Here's an important term I want to introduce you to: *nutrient-dense*. Nearly every morsel you put into your mouth will pack nutritional bang for your bite. If you were to eat 1 ounce of potato chips—that's about 10 chips, for the record—you would consume around 150 calories, but they'd be completely empty calories. Translation: Those greasy, deep-fried tubers would deliver *zero* nutrients to your body. Not only that, they would contribute a boatload of saturated fat—the kind that clogs arteries and promotes weight gain. A waste of 150 calories, wouldn't you say? Now consider what an apple and a spoonful of peanut butter provide with roughly the same amount of calories: *no* saturated fat, a bounty of nutrients, fiber, protein, and "good" monounsaturated fat. It's a simple switch, but one that will do endless good. Spotting a nutrient-dense food isn't even all that difficult, if you follow Glassman's three rules:

1. *Nutrient-dense starches and fruits* provide at least 3 grams of fiber per serving. Examples: black beans, brown rice, and raspberries.
2. *Nutrient-dense proteins* contain as many grams of lean protein as possible and typically have no more than 5 grams of fat per serving. Examples: skinless white meat chicken, tofu, pork tenderloin, and lean cuts of beef.
3. *Nutrient-dense fats* are high in mono- and polyunsaturated fats. They also have very few grams of saturated fats, contain no trans fats, and often have a beneficial ratio of omega-3 and omega-6 fatty acids. Examples: avocado, nuts, olive oil, flaxseed, and fish.

You Can Keep Your Social Life!

How often has "being on a diet" meant skipping an evening out with friends? The LBN plan allows for two drinks a week. You'll have to bypass the sugar- and calorie-heavy margaritas, of course, but you can have my signature LBN cocktail instead!

The Signature *Look Better Naked* **Cocktail**
When you're out, have a bartender shake
2 oz vodka, 1 oz St-Germain (an elderflower
liqueur), and ½ oz fresh lime juice with ice.
Strain or, if desired, add a splash of seltzer,
and garnish with fresh mint leaves.

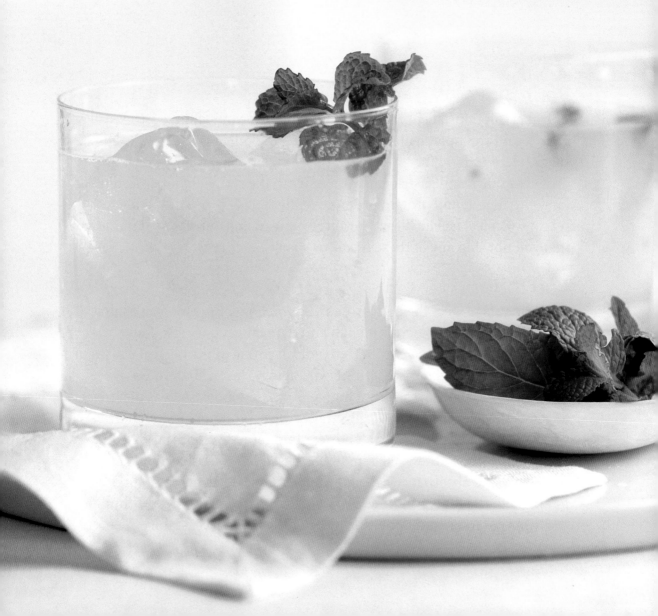

Quick and easy to prepare, the delicious meals in *Look Better Naked* will leave you feeling full, fire up your metabolism, and help you transform your body.

Your Belly Will Feel Full!

The fiber/protein/fat combo in that apple-and-peanut-butter snack will not only fill you up, it will also keep you feeling full longer than the chips snack. Here's why: Fiber-rich foods take longer to chew, and chewing produces saliva and gastric juices that fill up the stomach. Fiber also takes longer to digest, and protein promotes satiety. This is one of the biggest reasons you feel lackluster when you're hungry, and why it's so imperative that you not skip any of these meals or snacks.

You'll Bring Out Your Best!

Antioxidants protect the body from *free radicals*—rogue molecules that travel around your body raising hell and damaging your cells. Many experts believe that damage from free radicals is one of the biggest causes of cancer, cardiovascular disease, and even aging. Unfortunately, many realities of our daily lives—from highly processed foods such as deli meats to car exhaust and UV rays—help trigger the production of free radicals within our bodies. But certain foods contain more free-radical-fighting antioxidants than others. Glassman has based her food selections on the oxygen radical absorbance capacity, or ORAC, scale, which measures a food's potential for controlling free radicals. (As a general rule of thumb, the deeper, darker, and richer the color of the fruit or vegetable, the more antioxidants it contains.) Because many of the benefits of antioxidants are physically apparent ones—they'll ward off wrinkles, for example—these nutrients are abundant in the Look Better Naked diet.

You'll Feel Energized!

The LBN diet is designed to complement the LBN fitness plan, which begins on page 92. The foods will support and even maximize the gains from your workouts—including postgym snacks that contain optimal amounts of carbs and protein for muscle repair, such as almond butter on whole-grain crackers, and chocolate milk! Why the moo juice? Researchers have found that athletes who drink low-fat chocolate milk have muscle recovery equal to or better than that of athletes who have a sports drink containing the same number of calories. In a perfect world I'd like you to eat something at least an hour before your workouts and then have the designated post-workout snacks about 15 minutes after you're done.

I hope that you're no longer dreading this crucial element of the program. Hopefully you understand its effectiveness and, more important, its pleasure quotient. *Bon appetit!*

The Top 20 of LBN Foods

Avocados

This luscious fruit is famous for containing loads of cholesterol-lowering, heart-healthy monounsaturated fat, which boosts the "bioavailability" of antioxidants in foods that it's paired with. Tomatoes are an especially good complement—a fact that makes a strong case for adding tomatoes to your guacamole—because they're rich in lycopene, a pigment-rich antioxidant known as a carotenoid that reduces cancer risk and cardiovascular disease. To whip up your own avocado salad dressing, puree a medium avocado with 2 tablespoons of lemon juice and a dash of cayenne (both LBN guilt-free flavor boosters). If an avocado is firm, place it in a paper bag with an apple or banana, which will emit ripening ethylene gas. And if you're only going to eat half the avocado, leave the pit in the part you don't use; it will prevent browning.

Beef

Nothing beats pure protein when it comes to building muscle. The problem with most store-bought beef, however, is that the majority of cattle are fed grain, which gives their meat a relatively high ratio of omega-6 to omega-3 fatty acids. This, in turn, contributes to a host of problems. The fatty acids in grass-fed beef, on the other hand, are skewed toward the omega-3 variety. Such beef also contains conjugated linoleic acid (CLA), which studies have shown helps reduce belly fat and build lean muscle. Beef is also among the best sources of highly absorbable iron in your supermarket. Low iron levels, which are common in women, not only zap your zip, but can also cause brittle nails, according to Francesca Fusco, MD, an assistant clinical professor of dermatology at New York City's Mount Sinai Medical Center.

Berries

Take your pick—blackberries, blueberries, raspberries, and strawberries are all insanely good for you. In general, the darker the berry, the sweeter the juice—and the better it is for you. Blackberries, for instance, are loaded with anthocyanins, powerful antioxidant compounds that have been shown to improve brain function (and are also found in red wine and tea). Can't say anything bad about blueberries either, but wild varieties contain 26 percent more antioxidants than cultivated ones. Blueberries also contain vision-protecting vitamin C as well as appetite-quelling fiber (although raspberries have more fiber than any other berries). And scientists now believe that blueberries battle urinary tract infections, says Elizabeth Somer, RD. Strawberries pack up to three times more vitamin C than other berries and have fewer calories, but they're one of the most important foods to buy organic, according to Keith Block, MD, author of *Life Over Cancer*, because they have a unique capacity for absorbing pesticides.

Black Beans

Beans are a healthy way to add protein to your diet, as well as potassium, folate, and iron—and the darker the beans, the better,

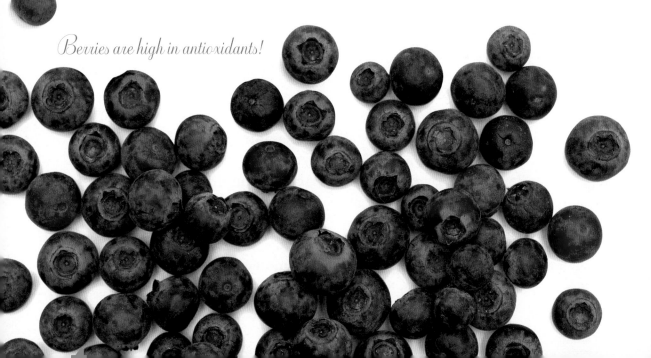

Berries are high in antioxidants!

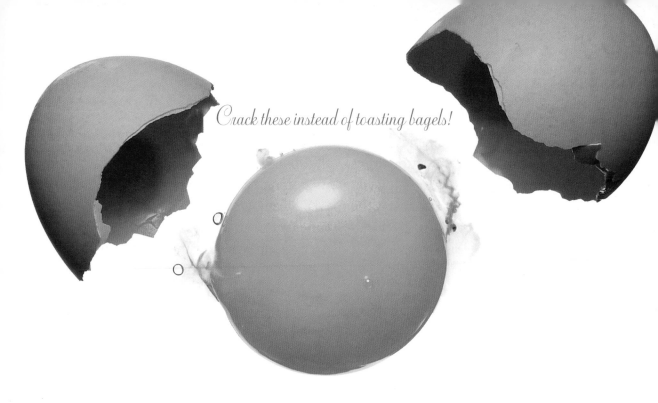

Crack these instead of toasting bagels!

concluded researchers at the University of Guelph in Ontario. Their study found that beans are loaded with the same heart-healthy, cancer-preventing compounds found in red wine, berries, and tea. But black beans had the most, followed by red, brown, yellow, and white. (For comparison's sake, ½ cup of black beans had the same amount of anthocyanins as two glasses of red wine.) But don't discount good-for-you yellow legumes, such as soybeans. All beans are low in fat, and they're packed with protein, fiber, and iron—nutrients crucial for building muscle and losing weight.

Bell Peppers

Bright-red peppers have high levels of antioxidant vitamins A and C, according to James O. Hill, PhD, director of the Center for Human Nutrition at the University of Colorado and co-founder of America on the Move, a national weight-gain-prevention initiative. Just 1 cup of chopped red peppers contains three times the minimum amount of vitamin C and nearly 100 percent of the vitamin A recommended for a typical 2,000-calorie-a-day diet. Green and yellow peppers contain less vitamin A, but all peppers are naturally fat free and low calorie, and they contain 3 grams of fiber per chopped cup, making them excellent snacks or mealtime fillers.

Brussels Sprouts

Selenium is a vital trace mineral that mops up those pesky free radicals and helps protect against heart disease, type 2 diabetes, and cancer, according to Matthew Kadey, RD. A cup of Brussels sprouts contains twice as much selenium as, say, butternut squash or kale. "Your thyroid can't produce certain hormones without it," he says. "You can blame hormones for a lot of bad stuff, but they also happen to run your entire system—and thyroid hormones, specifically, control the metabolism of every cell in your body." Plus the sulforaphane in Brussels sprouts fires up enzymes that may stop breast-cancer cells from growing.

Chicken Breast

In terms of lean protein, white meat chicken (minus the skin) reigns supreme. And lean protein is also a terrific source of coenzyme Q10, which assists skin cell turnover. (So goodbye flaky old dead cells, and hello fresh, rosy new ones!) You can easily grill enough chicken for a week's worth of meals—to chunk into salads or slice for sandwiches, for example. Just rub a pound of boneless, skinless chicken breasts with olive oil, garlic, and dried rosemary and fire on each side for about 5 minutes, and then store in the fridge for up to a week.

Dried Fruit

A San Diego State University study turned up this bit of fulfilling news about dried plums, aka prunes: They're supremely satiating. Women who ate 12 prunes one day, then ate the equivalent calories' worth of low-fat cookies the next day, said they felt significantly less hungry 2 hours after eating the fruit than they did after eating the cookies. The abundant fiber and sorbitol (a sugar alcohol that the body metabolizes slowly) in prunes keep blood sugar and insulin levels in check. Prunes may also help shrink your waistline. A study published in the *American Journal of Clinical Nutrition* found that among 74,000 women surveyed, those who got more fiber were 49 percent less likely to suffer weight gain. Prunes help fight the hardening of arteries and pack a powerful antioxidant punch, too. Dried cherries are another good option.

Eggs

The ideal breakfast, according to Larry McCleary, MD, author of *The Brain Trust Program,* is an egg. The incredible edible contains B vitamins, which enable nerve cells to burn glucose, your brain's major energy source; antioxidants, which protect neurons against damage; and omega-3 fatty acids, which keep nerve cells firing at optimal speed. They're good for your belly, too. Those who eat eggs for breakfast lose 65 percent more weight than those who eat a bagel breakfast with the same number of calories, according to a study in the *International Journal of Obesity.* Opt for Organic Valley Omega-3 eggs, which contain 225 milligrams of omega-3s.

Flaxseed

These super seeds have the highest levels of *lignans,* estrogen-like compounds known as phytoestrogens, of any food. In fact, women who eat the most lignans have the lowest body mass indexes. In research on animals, estrogen quells appetite and shrinks fat cells, and phytoestrogens may have a similar effect in people, says Anne-Sophie Morisset, RD, of Laval University in Quebec. Give the seeds a spin in your coffee grinder and sprinkle the grounds on cereal or yogurt, or blend them into smoothies. You can also find flaxseed in multigrain breads and cereals.

Hummus

This is now your official go-to dip instead of the calorie bomb that is ranch dressing (75 or more calories per tablespoon!). High in fiber and lower in saturated fat and calories, hummus pairs equally well with veggies. To make it, mix the following ingredients in a food processor until smooth and creamy: two 10-ounce cans garbanzo beans (chickpeas), drained, with ⅓ cup liquid reserved; juice of one lemon; 3 tablespoons olive oil; two garlic cloves; 1 teaspoon salt; 1 teaspoon ground cumin. Serve immediately, or cover and chill until ready to use.

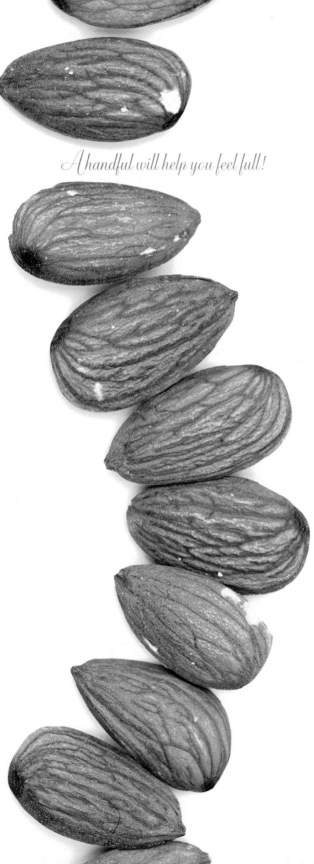

A handful will help you feel full!

Milk, Yogurt, & Cheese

Low-fat, calcium-rich foods can help you lose weight in the long term. A study in the *British Journal of Nutrition* found that obese women who doubled their daily intake of calcium from 600 milligrams per day to 1,200 milligrams over the course of 15 weeks lost an average of 11 pounds—without cutting calories! Plain low-fat yogurt, especially the Greek-style stuff, provides muscle-friendly protein and contains less sugar than other types. Reduced-fat cottage cheese is another protein heavyweight, with 14 grams in half a cup. In addition to building muscle, calcium will help you attain a strong, vibrant mane, because hair is almost all protein.

Nuts & Nut Butters

To get moist, beautiful, chap-free lips, your body needs to constantly replace old skin cells with new ones. Reach for walnuts. "Their omega-3 fats help regulate this turnover so that it happens all the time," says Fusco. Almonds are bursting with vitamin E, an antioxidant that bolsters the immune system, and almond butter is an easy flavor upgrade from peanut butter. A 2007 Penn State study also found that eating 1½ ounces of pistachios a day lowers blood pressure.

Olives & Extra-Virgin Olive Oil

A single tablespoon of olive oil delivers 10 grams of monounsaturated fat. Adding olive oil to red, green, orange, or yellow fruits and vegetables increases the amount of heart-saving, cancer-fighting, vision-boosting, immune-repairing, bone-strengthening vitamins such as A, E, and K, as well as carotenoids. For a quick salad dressing, pair two parts olive oil with one part antioxidant-rich balsamic vinegar, which can improve vascular function.

Salmon

Eat wild salmon from Alaska and you'll be taking advantage of a nutritional all-star. Not only can this tasty fish's omega-3 fatty acids lower bad cholesterol and boost your mood, it's also a great source of lean protein. NFL surveys suggest that many teams—including the Cincinnati Bengals and the New York Giants—serve it to players to lock in strength gains and fuel performance. You won't need to eat nearly as much as a football player, but here's another reason to love it: Eating salmon helps your body produce wrinkle-fighting friends, such as collagen and keratin. Yet another score!

Tofu

Made from pressed soybean curds, tofu was once the bastion of vegetarians. But the plant protein in tofu—which comes in firm or soft varieties, and is delicious marinated and tossed in salads—provides a full complement of amino acids, as well as isoflavone, which helps muscles recover from exercise.

Tuna

Tuna is one of the best sources of lean protein, but instead of mixing in a lot of mayo and turning it into a fatty disaster, add pepper, hot sauce, and some fresh lemon juice. Or toss some chunk light into your salads. A 3-ounce serving contains 11 mg of heart-healthy niacin, which has been shown to help lower cholesterol and help your body process fat.

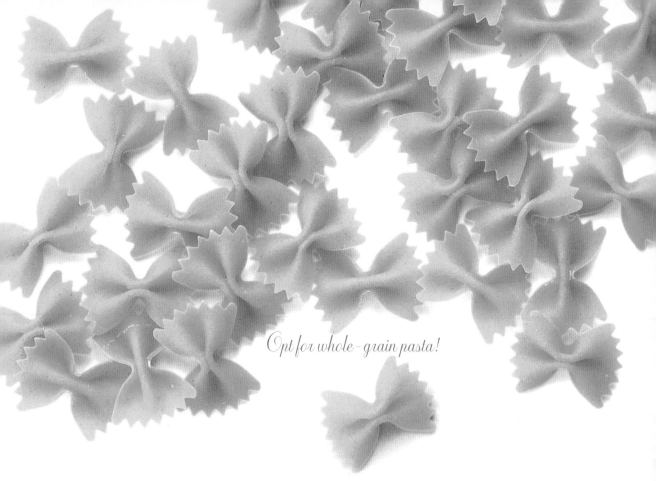

Opt for whole-grain pasta!

Researchers at the University of Rochester in New York determined that niacin raises HDL cholesterol (the good kind) and lowers triglycerides more than most cholesterol-lowering drugs alone.

Whole Grains

Oatmeal, wheat flour, barley, brown rice, and whole-grain sourdough bread are all high in fiber, which will keep you full by taking a long time to digest. Not all breads and crackers advertised as "whole grain" are the real deal, however. "Read the label," says Lynn Grieger, an online health, food, and fitness coach. "Those that aren't whole grain can be high in fat." Two easy options: Quaker Old-Fashioned Oats or The Baker Bread's seven-grain sourdough whole-wheat bread. Beginning your day with oats protects against diabetes, insulin resistance, and obesity, and researchers have found that sourdough causes less of a spike in blood sugar than any other type of bread.

guilt-free
Flavor boosters

▶▶ Think of this as a list of ingredients to get creative with.
Add the Moroccan spice mix to plain yogurt and use it as a sweet-
potato topping, for instance, or build a dressing for bok choy
out of lemon juice, garlic, and ginger. Use as much as you want!

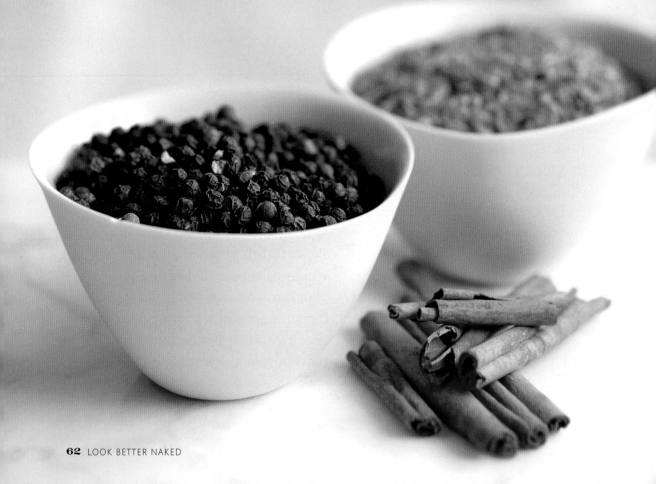

ingredients

- Dijon mustard
- Dried spices (any, such as basil, cinnamon, oregano)
- Fat-free low-sodium chicken broth
- Fresh ginger
- Fresh herbs
- Garlic
- Hot pepper flakes
- Lemon juice
- Lime juice
- Low-sodium soy sauce
- Pepper
- Salsa
- Vinegars (balsamic, red wine, flavored)
- White horseradish
- Worcestershire sauce

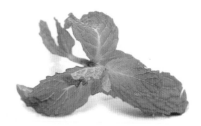

Here are some recommended combinations:

Greek:
¼ tsp dried oregano
¼ tsp dried mint
¼ tsp dried thyme
⅛ tsp dried basil
⅛ tsp dried marjoram
⅛ tsp dried parsley
⅛ tsp dried minced onion
⅛ tsp dried minced garlic

Spanish:
1 tsp garlic powder
1 tsp onion powder
1 tsp black pepper
¼ tsp oregano
¼ tsp chili powder
¼ tsp cumin

Italian:
Minced garlic to taste
½ tsp dried basil
¼ tsp dried thyme
¼ tsp dried rosemary
⅛ tsp crushed red pepper

Moroccan:
1 tsp ground cinnamon
1 tsp ground coriander
½ tsp ground turmeric
¼ tsp cayenne pepper
¼ tsp ground cardamom
¼ tsp ground cumin

Thai:
2 Tbsp lime juice
½ stalk of lemongrass (peeled and minced)
1 Tbsp minced fresh ginger
1 tsp Asian fish sauce

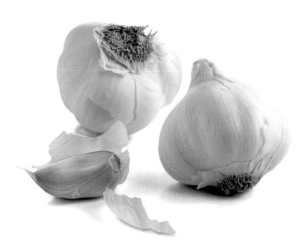

the *Little-bit-Naughty Flavor boosters*

➤➤ These flavor boosters are slightly more sinful than the guilt-free ones because they contain more sugar, more fat, or more calories. Limit yourself to two per day.

yogurt-based dips and marinades

- ¼ cup plain fat-free Greek yogurt,
  1 tsp cinnamon,
  1 tsp nutmeg
  For fruit.

- ¼ cup plain fat-free Greek yogurt ,
  1 Tbsp Dijon mustard
  As a dip or marinade for chicken, pork, or vegetables.

- ¾ cup plain fat-free Greek yogurt;
  1 crushed garlic clove;
  ¼ peeled, sliced cucumber; and
  2 tsp chopped fresh mint
  For chicken and vegetables.

- ½ cup plain fat-free Greek yogurt;
  1 sliced, peeled cucumber;
  ½ diced jalapeno;
  juice of ½ lime; and
  salt and pepper to taste
  Use 2 tablespoons with fish and chicken.

- ¼ cup plain fat-free Greek yogurt,
  1 tsp dill, and
  ¼ avocado
  For chicken and vegetables.

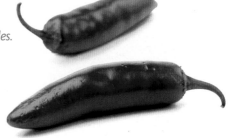

ingredients

- **1 Tbsp honey**
  Stir it into yogurt or oatmeal.

- **1 Tbsp ketchup**
  Add a dollop on a baked sweet potato or turkey burger.

- **1 Tbsp barbecue sauce**
  Pair with chicken or pork.

- **½ cup marinara sauce**
  Serve atop chicken or pasta, or as a dip for mozzarella cheese sticks.

- **Cottage cheese dip:**
  ½ cup nonfat cottage cheese, 1 Tbsp white horseradish, and black pepper; or ¼ cup nonfat cottage cheese mixed with 1 Tbsp salsa
  Serve with vegetables.

- **1 Tbsp chopped nuts**
  Toss into salads or sprinkle on fish.

- **3 Tbsp Parmesan cheese**
  Sprinkle on popcorn, salad, or veggies.

- **3 Tbsp cocoa powder**
  Blend it into a shake or pair with fruit.

- **3 Tbsp shredded coconut**
  Mix into salads or eat with fruit.

- **2 Tbsp chutney**
  Dollop onto pork or chicken.

- **2 Tbsp guacamole**
  Use as a dip for vegetables or add to soups or salads.

- **2 Tbsp mango salsa:** Mix 1 peeled, diced mango with ¼ small diced red onion, and 1 Tbsp chopped cilantro
  Pair with fish.

the *look better naked*

2-day cleanse

(a simple meal plan that will hit your body's reset button!)

➡ What are you doing this weekend? Ready to look better naked? Ideally, I'd like you to use this 2-day kick-start plan on Saturday and Sunday, and then begin the full fitness and diet plan the following Monday. It's purely optional, but the best way to get into the groove of a new approach to eating is by experiencing early results—a strategy that's worked over and over for hundreds of dietitian Keri Glassman's clients. The sooner you start looking and feeling better, the more motivated you will be to stick with the plan. That's why these 2 days of meals offer up less variety—but no less flavor—than the rest of the diet, and why they're a little lower in calories. You won't feel deprived or hungry, and you'll definitely have an overall feeling of well-being after going without processed foods, salt, and sugar. You'll feel healthy, and the drop in sodium alone will help you shed a little water weight.

It's important to eat exactly what's listed below on both days of the cleanse—but note that there's more variety here than meets the eye in terms of which foods you choose to eat and how you prepare them.

Breakfast

Light shake:
Blend 1 cup fat-free (or soy, almond, rice, or hemp) milk, 1 cup berries, 1 tsp peanut butter or flaxseed oil, and 1 cup of ice until frothy.

Bonus: Add a dash of cocoa powder!

Snack

1 cup sliced cucumbers
1 cup green tea

Bonus: Add a little vinegar and fresh dill to your cucumbers, or make a cucumber salad by slicing a couple of unpeeled cucumbers into rounds, dousing them with flavored vinegar (fig is great, if you can find it), and letting them marinate for an hour. Drain off the vinegar and keep them in the fridge.

Bonus: Drink your green tea straight up and hot—or brew a whole pot, toss in some fresh mint leaves or slices of peeled fresh ginger, and let steep for a few hours. Store in the fridge and pour it over ice when you're thirsty.

Lunch

Steamed or raw greens (romaine, spinach, mesclun mix, bok choy, arugula, watercress, frisee, endive, etc.)
4 oz lean protein (white meat chicken, firm tofu, lean beef, fish)
2 tsp oil (olive, sunflower, walnut)

Bonus: Mix-and-match your greens! You can get a lot of no-cal flavor simply by adding arugula or watercress, both of which have a peppery kick. Or you can toss a handful of fresh basil, cilantro, or flat-leaf parsley in with salad greens for an extra jolt of flavor.

Snack

10 asparagus spears, blanched
1 cup green tea

Bonus: Dip the asparagus into fat-free yogurt swirled with Dijon mustard to taste.

Dinner

Steamed or raw greens
4 oz lean protein
2 tsp oil

Bonus: Be creative with your 2 teaspoons of oil, at both lunch and dinner. Whisk it with a teaspoon of vinegar and some herbs for vinaigrette; use it to sauté bite-size pieces of white-meat chicken, lean beef, tofu, or fish; or mix it with a flavor-booster spice mix to rub on chicken, beef, or fish before broiling or grilling.

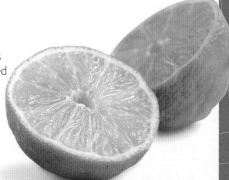

The LBN 6-Week Diet

The Look Better Naked eating plan is designed for flexibility and experimentation. Meals are interchangeable from day to day. Stick to the ingredients and amounts indicated in each—but feel free to play around with the flavor boosters. The items in parentheses on the menu will help get you started.

week 1

	MONDAY	TUESDAY	WEDNESDAY
Breakfast	**High-Fiber Cereal** ¾ cup high-fiber cereal sprinkled with 1 Tbsp ground flaxseed, with 1 cup fat-free milk 1 small sliced banana	**Egg White Wrap** 3 scrambled egg whites topped with 1 oz reduced-fat Cheddar cheese, wrapped in small whole-wheat tortilla Small fat-free latte	**Veggie Omelet** 1 whole egg, 2 egg whites, spinach, tomatoes, and mushrooms 1 slice whole-wheat toast 1 cup fat-free milk
Snack	2 Tbsp guacamole 6 jicama slices or carrot sticks	1 hard-boiled egg 1 cup sugar snap peas	1 oz 50 percent reduced-fat Cheddar cheese 1 cup sliced red and yellow bell peppers
Lunch	**Chopped Chef's Salad** Romaine lettuce, cucumbers, tomatoes, 2 egg whites, 3 oz turkey, and 1 oz reduced-fat Cheddar cheese tossed with 2 tsp olive oil (vinegar)	**Tuna Salad Pita** 1 can (4 oz) chunk light tuna packed in water, drained and stuffed into ½ whole-wheat pita with lettuce and tomatoes. Drizzle with lemon juice and 1 tsp olive oil.	**Chicken Lettuce Wrap** 4 oz sliced grilled chicken in large lettuce leaf. Top with chopped bell pepper, artichoke hearts, and 1 oz part-skim mozzarella cheese. (honey mustard) 1 cup raspberries
Post-Workout Snack	2 slices turkey on small whole-wheat wrap (guacamole)	**Trail Mix** 18 pistachios, 1 Tbsp dried cherries, ¼ cup oat bran flakes	100-calorie pack of microwave popcorn sprinkled with 2 Tbsp of Parmesan cheese
Dinner	**Grilled Steak** 4 oz beef tenderloin Steamed cauliflower, mashed with 2 Tbsp Parmesan cheese (chicken broth to help soften) Steamed green beans	**Baked Wild Salmon** 3 oz salmon, brushed with olive oil and baked, skin side down, for about 10 minutes at 425°F Steamed artichoke Mixed green salad with 1 Tbsp vinaigrette ½ cup quinoa	**Pork Tenderloin** 4 oz pork tenderloin seasoned with salt and pepper and roasted at 350°F for 15 minutes (paprika or Moroccan spice mix) Steamed green beans Spinach salad with sliced cherry tomatoes and red onions

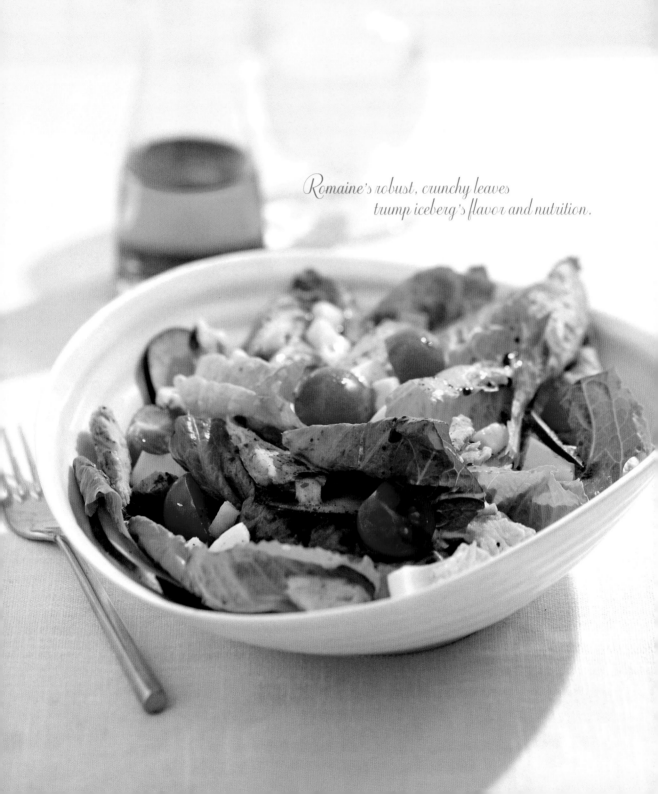

Romaine's robust, crunchy leaves trump iceberg's flavor and nutrition.

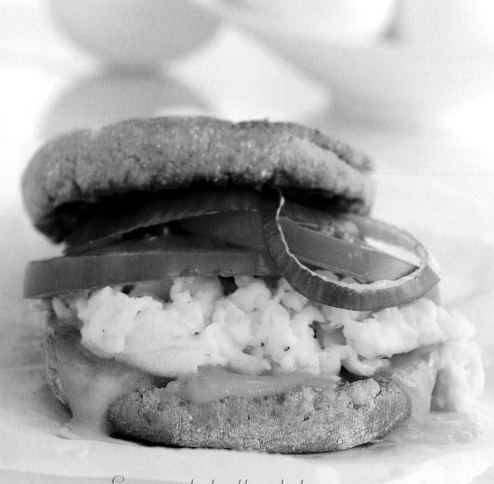

*Eating eggs for breakfast whittles
your middle and boosts your brainpower!*

How much are you *actually* eating?

A 1-ounce serving of cheese is about the same size as four dice or a Ping-Pong ball.

	THURSDAY	FRIDAY	SATURDAY	SUNDAY
Breakfast	**Yogurt Parfait** 1 cup nonfat plain yogurt with 1 Tbsp chopped almonds, 2 Tbsp wheat germ, and 1 cup diced mango	**PB Waffle** 1 whole-grain frozen waffle spread with 2 tsp natural peanut butter 1 cup fat-free milk 1 cup papaya	**Egg Sandwich** 1 whole-wheat English muffin topped with 2 scrambled egg whites, 2 slices tomato, 1 slice red onion, and 1 oz low-fat cheese 8 oz fat-free latte	**Apple Cinnamon Oatmeal** 1 packet plain instant oatmeal prepared with fat-free milk, topped with 7 chopped walnut halves, and 1 finely chopped apple (cinnamon)
Snack	½ cup nonfat cottage cheese ½ cup sliced zucchini (onion powder)	½ avocado (lemon juice)	½ cup steamed edamame (pepper)	18 pistachios 1 cup sliced cucumber
Lunch	**Soup and Salad** 1 cup black bean soup Mixed green salad with 1 Tbsp vinaigrette and 2 high-fiber crackers (2 Tbsp guacamole)	**Turkey-Guacamole Sandwich** 2 Tbsp hummus, 3 oz turkey, 2 Tbsp guacamole, and 1 tomato slice layered on 1 slice whole-grain bread	**Mediterranean Platter** 2 high-fiber crackers, 6 large olives, 4 Tbsp hummus, sliced cucumber, and red and yellow peppers 1 cup tomato soup	**Grilled Salmon Salad** 4 oz grilled salmon over romaine lettuce with 1 oz reduced-fat feta cheese, cherry tomatoes, and 1 Tbsp vinaigrette
Post-Workout Snack	2 fiber crackers 2 tsp almond butter (honey)	1 cup fat-free chocolate milk	**Sweet Shake** 1 cup fat-free milk, 1 cup ice, 2 tsp peanut butter, ½ banana, and 1 tsp cocoa powder (cinnamon, nutmeg)	Small whole-wheat wrap with sliced tomato and 1 Tbsp hummus
Dinner	**Shrimp and Linguine** 5 medium shrimp (sautéed, baked, or grilled), tossed with ½ cup whole-wheat pasta (any style), and 2 tsp olive oil Steamed broccoli (2 Tbsp grated Parmesan cheese)	**Grilled Chicken** 4 oz boneless, skinless chicken breast Steamed asparagus Mixed green salad with 1 Tbsp vinaigrette	**Grilled Chicken Sausage** 1 chicken sausage on salad of baby spinach, 1 oz reduced-fat feta cheese, and balsamic vinegar	**Pan-Cooked Tilapia** 4 oz tilapia cooked 2 to 3 minutes per side (Spanish spice mix and served with mango salsa) Roasted Brussels sprouts Mixed green salad with 2 tsp vinaigrette Small baked sweet potato (honey, nutmeg, cinnamon)

How much are you *actually* eating?

A slice of bread should be about the size of a CD case and as thick as a finger.

week 2

	MONDAY	TUESDAY	WEDNESDAY
Breakfast	**Breakfast Pizza** 1 whole-wheat English muffin topped with tomato slice and 1 oz reduced-fat Cheddar cheese. Heat until cheese melts. 1 cup fat-free milk	**Greek Wrap** 3 egg whites scrambled with chopped tomatoes and spinach and rolled up in whole-wheat tortilla with 1 oz crumbled reduced-fat feta cheese	**Smoked Salmon Sandwich** 1 toasted whole-wheat English muffin spread with ½ cup whipped cottage cheese and topped with 2 oz smoked salmon
Snack	8 pecan halves 2 dried figs	15 tamari almonds	15 walnut halves
Lunch	**Hummus Sandwich** ½ whole-wheat pita spread with 4 Tbsp hummus and filled with cucumber, tomato, alfalfa sprouts, and baby spinach 4 olives	**Antipasto Platter** 2 high-fiber crackers, 4 oz lean ham, 1 oz cubed part-skim mozzarella cheese, grilled eggplant, zucchini, and asparagus	**Open-Faced Veggie Sandwich** Grilled zucchini, eggplant, roasted peppers, artichoke hearts, and 1 oz part-skim mozzarella cheese layered on 1 slice whole-grain bread (balsamic vinegar)
Post-Workout Snack	**Sweet-Potato Chips** 1 small sweet potato, thinly sliced and placed on baking sheet coated with cooking spray; sprinkle with sea salt and bake at 375°F for 25 minutes, or until crispy	1 medium apple 2 tsp peanut butter	**Tart Shake** 1 cup nonfat plain Greek yogurt, 1 cup ice, ½ cup frozen unsweetened cherries, and 1 Tbsp flaxseed (2 mint leaves)
Dinner	**Asian Stir Fry** 4 oz firm tofu, drained and cubed, sautéed with bok choy in 2 tsp olive oil and topped with 1 Tbsp sesame seeds Mixed green salad with 1 Tbsp vinaigrette	**Seared Sea Scallops** 5 large scallops, onion, garlic, and bell peppers seared in 2 tsp olive oil (red pepper flakes) ⅓ cup brown rice	**Grilled Bison Steak** 4 oz bison steak Broccoli Spinach salad with 1 oz goat cheese

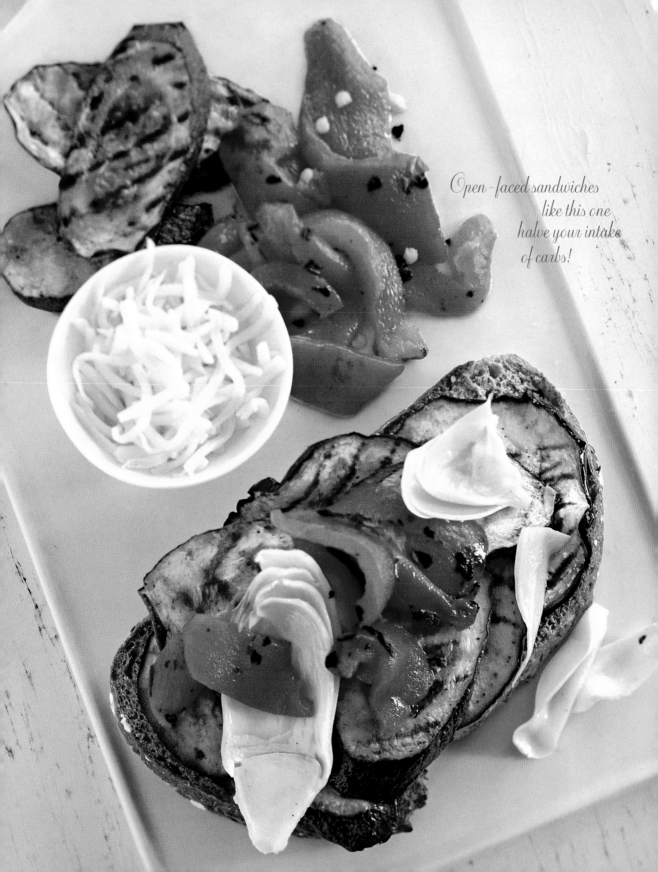

Open-faced sandwiches like this one halve your intake of carbs!

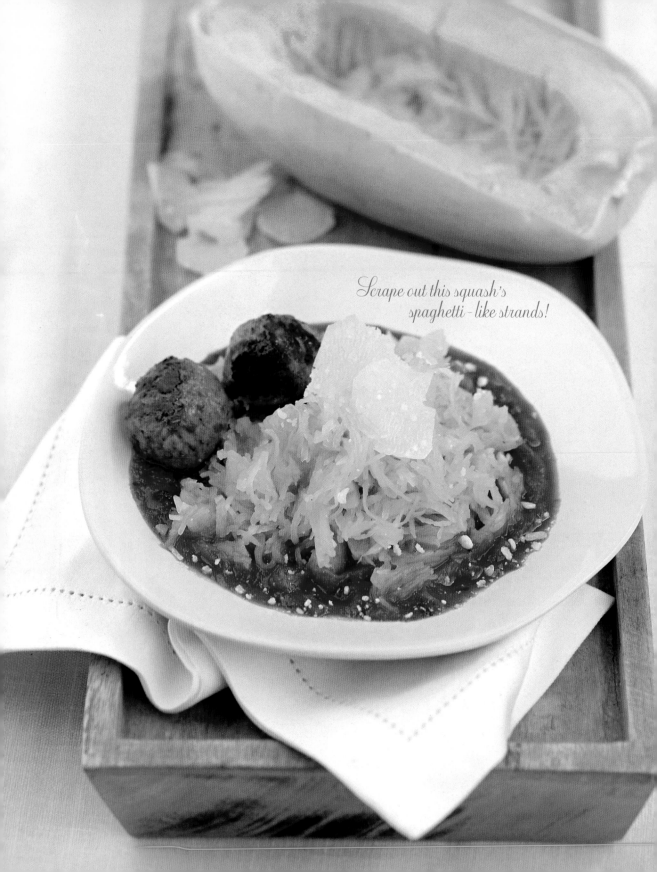

*Scrape out this squash's
spaghetti-like strands!*

A serving of marinara sauce is about the size of three whole eggs.

week 2
continued

	THURSDAY	FRIDAY	SATURDAY	SUNDAY
Breakfast	**French Toast** 1 slice whole-wheat bread soaked in 1 beaten egg and cooked in small skillet coated with nonstick cooking spray 1 cup fat-free milk 1 cup blackberries	**Muesli** ⅓ cup rolled oats, 1 Tbsp wheat germ, 5 chopped almonds, and 3 chopped dried apricots served over ¾ cup fat-free plain yogurt	**Hearty Cereal:** ¾ cup oat bran flakes, 1 cup fat-free milk, and 1 Tbsp chopped pecans	**Broiled Grapefruit:** ½ grapefruit sprinkled with cinnamon and broiled until top is bubbly; serve with 1 slice whole-wheat toast spread with 2 tsp almond butter. 1 cup fat-free milk
Snack	1 oz herbed goat cheese spread on endive leaves	2 tsp coconut butter 2 fiber crackers	15 grapes ½ oz Parmesan cheese	1 cup cubed cantaloupe ½ cup fat-free cottage cheese
Lunch	**Pasta Salad** ½ cup whole-wheat pasta, steamed asparagus tips, 4 oz shrimp, and 2 Tbsp Parmesan cheese tossed with ½ cup marinara sauce	**Veggie Burger** 1 veggie burger and ¼ of an avocado, sliced, on toasted whole-wheat English muffin (salsa) Mixed green salad (lemon juice or vinegar)	**Asian Chicken Salad** 4 oz grilled chicken, 15 peanuts, sliced water chestnuts, carrots, scallions, and cucumber tossed with 2 tsp sesame oil and brown rice vinegar	**"Chicken Wing" Salad** 4 oz grilled chicken breast (hot sauce) and 1 Tbsp crumbled blue cheese tossed with romaine lettuce, carrots, celery, and 1 Tbsp vinaigrette
Post-Workout Snack	¾ cup fat-free plain Greek yogurt 1 Tbsp cocoa powder (cinnamon)	½ cup black bean dip Celery sticks	1 Tbsp chopped walnuts 1 cup raspberries	¾ cup fat-free plain Greek yogurt 3 Tbsp wheat germ (honey)
Dinner	**Poached Halibut** In a deep skillet, bring 4 cups water to a simmer with 3 thin slices of lemon. Gently add 4 oz halibut fillet (add more water if not covered by liquid) until the fish is opaque, about 10 minutes. (pepper, lemon, olive oil) Kale (2 tsp olive oil and sea salt), roasted until crispy Steamed carrots	**Turkey Burger** 4 oz ground turkey formed into a burger patty and served on whole-wheat English muffin (pepper, fresh herbs, dried spices, ketchup, Worcestershire sauce) 1 slice reduced-fat cheese Beet chips Arugula and tomato salad with 2 tsp vinaigrette	**Shrimp Kabobs** Skewer 5 medium shrimp, brush with 1 tsp olive oil, and grill over high heat for about 5 minutes, turning as they char. (lemon, pepper) ⅓ cup brown rice Snow peas Mixed green salad with 1 Tbsp vinaigrette	**Spaghetti Squash** 1 spaghetti squash, halved and seeds removed; microwave (cut side up, covered with plastic wrap) for 12 minutes and scrape out flesh with a fork. Mix with marinara sauce, 2 Tbsp Parmesan cheese, and 3 small turkey meatballs.

How much are you *actually* eating?

A pinch of a spice measures
⅛ teaspoon, and a dash is
the equivalent to ¹⁄₁₆ teaspoon.

week 3

	MONDAY	TUESDAY	WEDNESDAY
Breakfast	**Yogurt Parfait** ¾ cup fat-free plain yogurt with 1 Tbsp chopped almonds, and 2 Tbsp wheat germ 1 cup berries	**Egg White Wrap** 3 scrambled egg whites, topped with 1 oz reduced fat Cheddar cheese, wrapped in small whole-wheat tortilla Small fat-free latte	**French Toast** 1 slice whole-wheat bread soaked in 1 beaten egg and cooked in small skillet coated with nonstick cooking spray 1 cup blackberries
Snack	1 oz herbed goat cheese spread onto endive	½ avocado (lemon juice)	2 fiber crackers 2 tsp almond butter (honey)
Lunch	**Chopped Chef's Salad** Romaine lettuce, cucumbers, tomatoes, 2 egg whites, 2 oz turkey, and 1 oz reduced-fat Cheddar cheese with 1 tsp olive oil and vinegar	**Tuna Salad Pita** 1 can (6 oz) chunk light tuna packed in water, drained and placed in ½ whole-wheat pita with lettuce and tomatoes, drizzled with lemon juice and 2 tsp olive oil	**Grilled Chicken Salad** 4 oz grilled salmon over romaine lettuce with 1 oz reduced-fat feta cheese, cherry tomatoes, and 1 Tbsp vinaigrette
Post-Workout Snack	**Sweet Shake** 1 cup fat-free milk 1 cup ice, 2 tsp peanut butter, ½ banana, and 1 tsp cocoa powder (cinnamon, nutmeg)	1 apple 2 tsp peanut butter	1 small whole-wheat wrap with sliced tomato and 2 Tbsp hummus
Dinner	**Pork Tenderloin** 4 oz pork tenderloin seasoned with salt and pepper and roasted at 350°F for 15 minutes (paprika or Moroccan spice mix) Steamed green beans Spinach salad with sliced cherry tomatoes and red onions	**Grilled Chicken Sausage** 1 chicken sausage on salad of baby spinach, 1 oz reduced-fat feta cheese, and balsamic vinegar	**Poached Halibut** In a deep skillet, bring 4 cups water to a simmer with 3 thin slices of lemon. Gently add 4 oz halibut fillet (add more water if not covered by liquid) until the fish is opaque, about 10 minutes. (pepper, lemon, olive oil) Kale (2 tsp olive oil and sea salt), roasted until crispy Steamed carrots

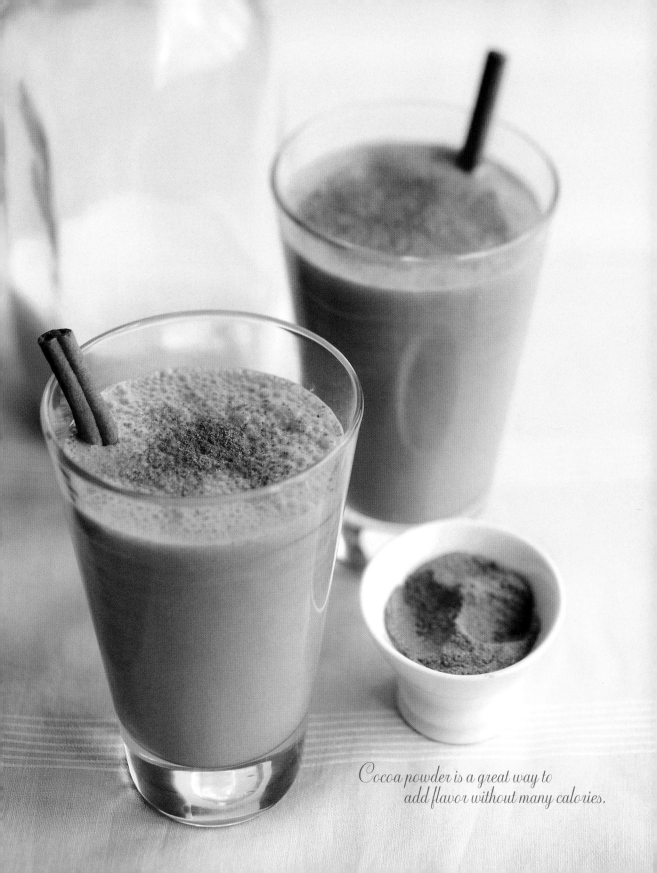

*Cocoa powder is a great way to
add flavor without many calories.*

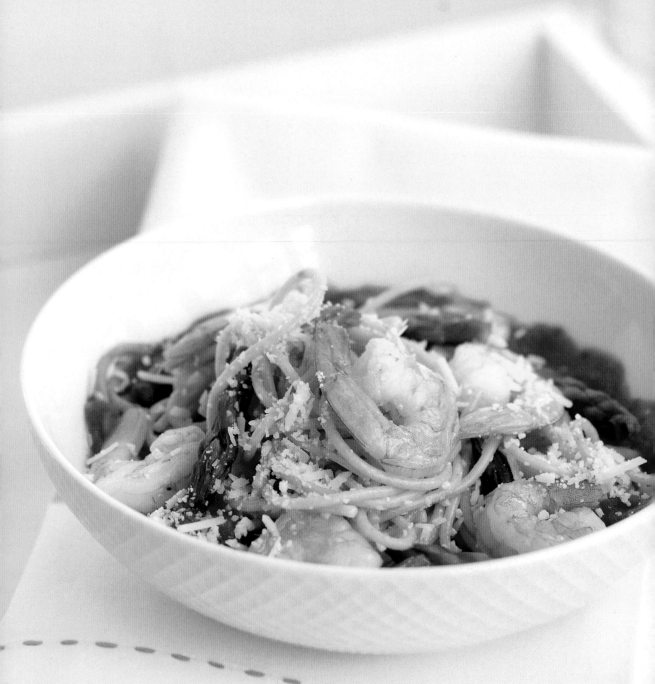

Shrimp, a low-fat source of protein, is also high in iron and zinc.

How much are you *actually* eating?

A ½-cup serving of cooked spaghetti is about the same size as your fist.

	THURSDAY	FRIDAY	SATURDAY	SUNDAY
Breakfast	**Apple Cinnamon Oatmeal** 1 packet plain instant oatmeal prepared with fat-free milk, with 7 chopped walnut halves and ½ of a finely chopped apple (cinnamon)	**Veggie Omelet** 1 whole egg, 2 egg whites, spinach, tomatoes, and mushrooms 1 slice whole-wheat toast 1 cup fat-free milk	**Greek Wrap** 3 egg whites scrambled with chopped tomatoes and spinach on whole-wheat tortilla, topped with 1 oz reduced-fat crumbled feta cheese	**PB Waffle** 1 whole-grain frozen waffle spread with 2 teaspoons natural peanut butter 1 cup fat-free milk
Snack	18 pistachios	15 walnut halves	1 hard-boiled egg	15 tamari almonds 1 apple
Lunch	**Open-Faced Veggie Sandwich** Grilled zucchini, eggplant, roasted peppers, artichoke hearts, and 1 oz part-skim mozzarella cheese over 1 slice whole-grain bread (balsamic vinegar)	**Hearty Soup** 1 cup black bean soup Mixed green salad with 2 tsp vinaigrette and 2 high-fiber crackers (guacamole)	**Pasta Salad** ½ cup whole-wheat pasta, steamed asparagus tips, 4 oz shrimp, 2 Tbsp Parmesan cheese (marinara sauce) 1 cup blackberries	**Hummus Sandwich** ½ whole-wheat pita, 2 Tbsp hummus, cucumber, tomato, alfalfa sprouts, and baby spinach 4 olives
Post-Workout Snack	¾ cup fat-free Greek yogurt 1 Tbsp cocoa powder (cinnamon)	1 cup pineapple 1 Tbsp chopped walnuts	100-calorie pack microwave popcorn sprinkled with 3 Tbsp Parmesan cheese	**Sweet-Potato Chips** 1 small sweet potato, thinly sliced and placed on baking sheet coated with cooking spray. Sprinkle with sea salt and bake at 375°F for 25 minutes, or until crispy.
Dinner	**Grilled Chicken** 4 oz boneless, skinless chicken breast Steamed asparagus Mixed green salad with 2 tsp vinaigrette Steamed carrots	**Pan-Cooked Tilapia** 4 oz tilapia cooked 2 to 3 minutes per side (Spanish spice mix and served with Mango salsa) Roasted brussels sprouts Mixed green salad with 2 tsp vinaigrette dressing Small baked sweet potato (honey, nutmeg, cinnamon)	**Turkey Burger** 4 oz ground turkey formed into a burger patty and served on whole-wheat English muffin (pepper, fresh herbs, dried spices, ketchup, Worcestershire sauce) 1 slice reduced-fat cheese Beet chips Arugula and tomato salad with 2 tsp vinaigrette	**Seared Sea Scallops** 5 large scallops, onion, garlic, and bell peppers seared in 2 tsp olive oil (red pepper flakes) ⅓ cup brown rice

How much are you *actually* eating?

A ½-cup serving of a fruit is about the same size as a lightbulb.

week 4

	MONDAY	TUESDAY	WEDNESDAY
Breakfast	**Smoked Salmon Sandwich** 1 toasted whole-wheat English muffin, spread with ½ cup whipped cottage cheese and topped with 2 oz smoked salmon	**Broiled Grapefruit** ½ grapefruit sprinkled with cinnamon, broiled until top is bubbly, and served with 1 slice whole-wheat toast and 2 tsp almond butter 1 cup fat-free milk	**Muesli** ⅓ cup rolled oats mixed with 1 Tbsp wheat germ, 5 chopped almonds, and 3 chopped dried apricots served over ¾ cup fat-free plain yogurt
Snack	8 pecan halves 2 dried figs	2 tsp coconut butter 2 fiber crackers	**Trail Mix** 18 pistachios, 1 Tbsp dried cherries, and ¼ cup oat bran flakes
Lunch	**Asian Chicken Salad** 4 oz grilled chicken, 15 peanuts, sliced water chestnuts, carrots, scallions, and cucumber tossed with 2 tsp sesame oil and brown rice vinegar	**Chicken Lettuce Wrap** 4 oz sliced, grilled chicken in large lettuce leaf topped with chopped bell pepper, artichoke hearts, and 1 oz part-skim mozzarella cheese (honey mustard)	**Chopped Chef's Salad** Romaine lettuce, cucumbers, tomatoes, 2 egg whites, 3 oz turkey, and 1 oz reduced-fat Cheddar cheese tossed with 2 tsp olive oil
Post-Workout Snack	½ cup black bean dip Celery sticks	2 Tbsp hummus on small whole-wheat wrap with sliced tomato	¾ cup fat-free plain Greek yogurt 3 Tbsp wheat germ (honey)
Dinner	**Shrimp Kabobs** Skewer 5 medium shrimp, brush with 1 tsp olive oil, and grill over high heat for about 5 minutes, turning as they char Snow peas Mixed green salad with 1 Tbsp vinaigrette ⅓ cup brown rice	**Asian Stir Fry** 4 oz firm tofu, drained and cubed, sautéed with bok choy in 2 tsp olive oil and topped with 1 Tbsp sesame seeds Mixed green salad with 1 Tbsp vinaigrette	**Spaghetti Squash** 1 spaghetti squash, halved and seeds removed; microwave (cut side up, covered with plastic wrap) for 12 minutes and scrape out flesh with a fork. Mix with marinara sauce, 2 Tbsp Parmesan cheese, and 3 small turkey meatballs.

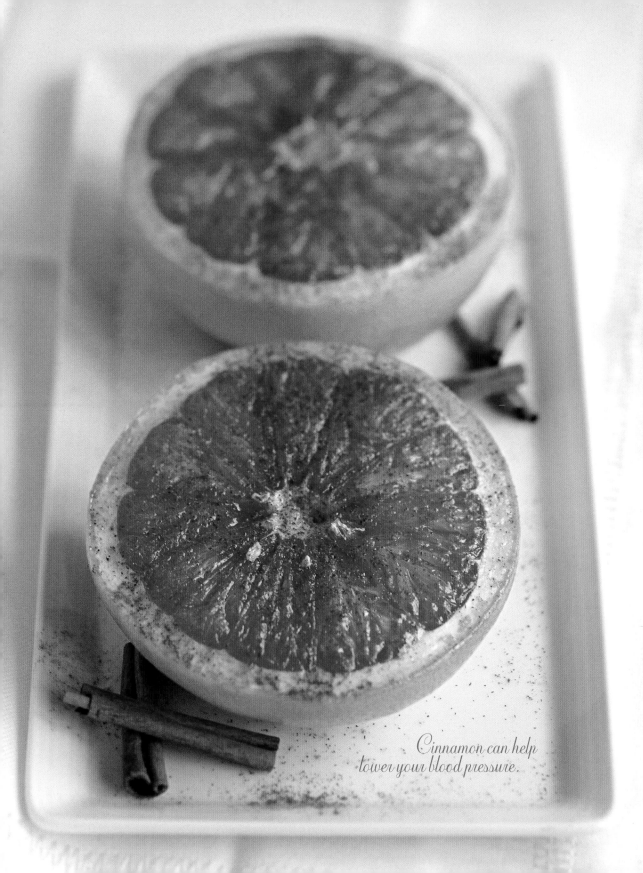

*Cinnamon can help
lower your blood pressure.*

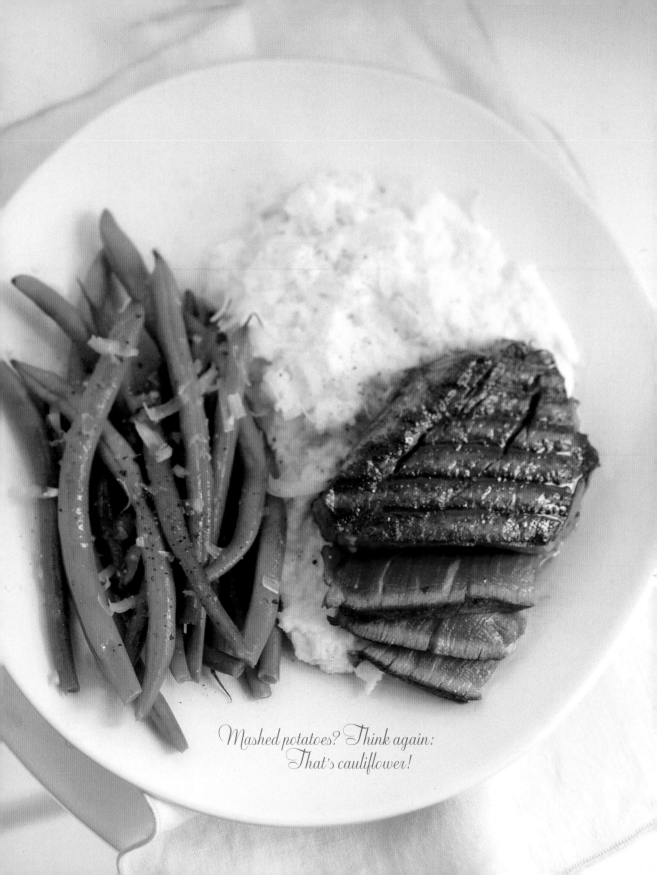

Mashed potatoes? Think again:
That's cauliflower!

A 4-ounce serving of beef is slightly larger than a deck of playing cards.

week 4
continued

	THURSDAY	FRIDAY	SATURDAY	SUNDAY
Breakfast	**High-Fiber Cereal** ¾ cup high-fiber cereal sprinkled with 1 Tbsp ground flaxseed, with 1 cup fat-free milk 1 small sliced banana	**Breakfast Pizza** 1 whole-wheat English muffin topped with tomato slice and 1 oz reduced-fat Cheddar cheese, heated until cheese melts 1 cup fat-free milk	**Hearty Cereal** ¾ cup oat bran flakes, 1 cup fat-free milk, 1 Tbsp chopped macadamia nuts, and 1 cup raspberries	**Egg Sandwich** 1 whole-wheat English muffin topped with 2 scrambled egg whites, 2 slices tomatoes, and 1 slice red onion 8 oz fat-free latte
Snack	1 cup cubed cantaloupe ½ cup nonfat cottage cheese	1 oz 50 percent reduced-fat Cheddar cheese Sliced red and bell yellow peppers	1 Tbsp guacamole 6 jicama slices or carrot sticks	1 cup steamed edamame (pepper)
Lunch	**Turkey Guacamole Sandwich** Open-faced sandwich made with 2 Tbsp hummus, 2 oz turkey, 2 Tbsp guacamole, and 1 tomato slice on 1 slice whole-grain bread	**"Chicken Wing" Salad** 4 oz grilled chicken breast (hot sauce) and 1 Tbsp crumbled blue cheese tossed with romaine lettuce, carrots, celery, and 1 Tbsp vinaigrette	**Veggie Burger** Veggie burger and ¼ of an avocado, sliced, on toasted English muffin (salsa) Mixed green salad (lemon juice or vinegar)	**Mediterranean Platter** 2 high-fiber crackers, 6 large olives, 4 Tbsp hummus, and sliced cucumber and red and yellow bell peppers
Post-Workout Snack	2 fiber crackers 2 tsp almond butter (honey)	**Tart Shake** 1 cup nonfat plain Greek yogurt, 1 cup ice, ½ cup frozen unsweetened cherries, and 1 Tbsp flaxseed (2 mint leaves)	2 slices turkey on small whole-wheat wrap (guacamole)	**Sweet Shake** 1 cup fat-free milk, 1 cup ice, 2 tsp peanut butter, ½ banana, and 1 tsp cocoa powder (cinnamon, nutmeg)
Dinner	**Grilled Bison Steak** 4 oz bison steak Broccoli Spinach salad with 1 oz goat cheese	**Shrimp and Linguine** 5 medium shrimp (sautéed, baked, or grilled), tossed with ½ cup whole-wheat pasta (any style), and 2 tsp olive oil Steamed broccoli (2 Tbsp grated Parmesan cheese)	**Grilled Steak** 4 oz beef tenderloin Steamed cauliflower, mashed with 2 Tbsp Parmesan cheese (chicken broth to help soften) Steamed green beans	**Seared Sea Scallops** 5 large scallops, onion, garlic, and bell peppers seared in 2 tsp olive oil (red pepper flakes) ⅓ cup brown rice

A ½-cup serving of vegetables is about the same size as a small yogurt container.

week 5

	MONDAY	TUESDAY	WEDNESDAY
Breakfast	**Veggie Omelet** 1 whole egg, 2 egg whites, spinach, tomatoes, and mushrooms 1 slice whole-wheat toast 1 cup fat-free milk	**High-Fiber Cereal** ¾ cup high-fiber cereal with 2 Tbsp ground flaxseed and 1 cup fat-free milk 1 small sliced banana	**Greek Wrap** 3 egg whites scrambled with chopped tomatoes and spinach, topped with 1 oz crumbled reduced-fat feta cheese and wrapped in whole-wheat tortilla
Snack	½ of an avocado (lemon juice)	18 pistachios 1 cup sliced cucumbers	8 pecan halves 2 dried figs
Lunch	**Open-Faced Veggie Sandwich** Grilled zucchini, eggplant, roasted peppers, artichoke hearts, and 1 oz part-skim mozzarella cheese over 1 slice whole-grain bread (balsamic vinegar)	**Turkey Guacamole Sandwich** Open-faced sandwich made with 2 Tbsp hummus, 2 oz turkey, 2 Tbsp guacamole, and 1 tomato slice on 1 slice whole-grain bread	**Pasta Salad** ½ cup whole-wheat pasta, steamed asparagus tips, 4 oz shrimp, and 2 Tbsp Parmesan cheese tossed with ½ cup marinara sauce
Post-Workout Snack	1 apple 2 tsp peanut butter	½ cup black bean dip Celery sticks	1 cup fat-free chocolate milk 8 almonds
Dinner	**Poached Halibut** In a deep skillet, bring 4 cups water to a simmer with 3 thin slices of lemon. Gently add 4 oz halibut fillet (add more water if not covered by liquid) until the fish is opaque, about 10 minutes. (pepper, lemon, olive oil) Kale (2 tsp olive oil and sea salt), roasted until crispy Steamed carrots	**Grilled Chicken Sausage** 1 chicken sausage on salad of baby spinach, 1 oz reduced-fat feta cheese, and balsamic vinegar	**Shrimp Kabobs** Skewer 5 medium shrimp, brush with 1 tsp olive oil, and grill over high heat for about 5 minutes, turning as they char. (lemon, pepper) Snow peas Mixed greens with 1 Tbsp vinaigrette

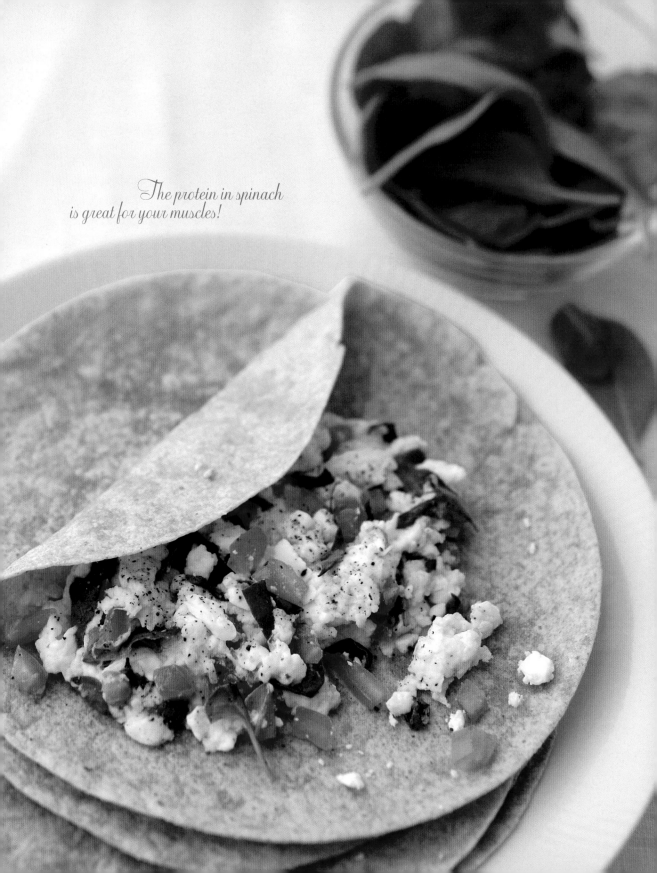

The protein in spinach is great for your muscles!

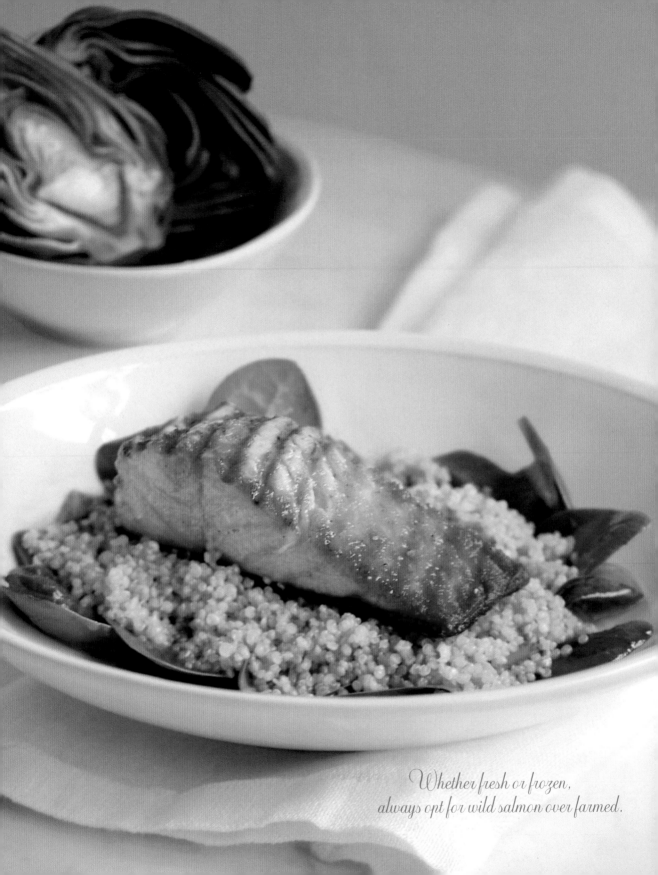

Whether fresh or frozen,
always opt for wild salmon over farmed.

How much are you *actually* eating?

A 3-ounce serving of fish is about the size of a checkbook.

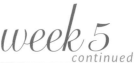

week 5
continued

	THURSDAY	FRIDAY	SATURDAY	SUNDAY
Breakfast	**Breakfast Pizza** 1 whole-wheat English muffin topped with tomato slice and 1 oz reduced-fat Cheddar cheese, heated until cheese melts 1 cup fat-free milk	**Egg Sandwich** 1 whole-wheat English muffin topped with 2 scrambled egg whites, 2 slices tomato, and 1 slice red onion 8 oz fat-free latte	**Yogurt Parfait** ¾ cup fat-free plain yogurt with 1 Tbsp chopped almonds, and 2 Tbsp wheat germ 1 cup berries	**French Toast** 1 slice whole-wheat bread soaked in 1 beaten egg and cooked in small skillet coated with nonstick cooking spray 1 cup blackberries
Snack	**Trail Mix** 18 pistachios, 1 Tbsp dried cherries, and ¼ cup oat bran flakes	1 cup cubed cantaloupe ½ cup nonfat cottage cheese	2 fiber crackers 2 tsp almond butter (honey)	15 walnut halves
Lunch	**Tuna Salad Pita:** 1 can (6-oz) chunk light tuna packed in water, drained and placed in ½ whole-wheat pita with lettuce and tomatoes, drizzled with lemon juice and 2 tsp olive oil	**Chopped Chef's Salad** Romaine lettuce, cucumbers, tomatoes, 2 egg whites, 2 oz turkey, 1 oz reduced-fat Cheddar cheese with 1 tsp olive oil and vinegar	**Hummus Sandwich** ½ whole-wheat pita spread with 2 Tbsp hummus and filled with cucumber, tomato, alfalfa sprouts, and baby spinach 4 olives	**Antipasto Platter** 2 high-fiber crackers, 2 oz lean ham, 1 oz cubed part-skim mozzarella cheese, grilled eggplant, zucchini, and asparagus
Post-Workout Snack	2 Tbsp hummus on small whole-wheat wrap with sliced tomato	1 cup pineapple 1 Tbsp chopped walnuts	¾ cup nonfat plain Greek yogurt 1 Tbsp cocoa powder (cinnamon)	2 fiber crackers 2 tsp almond butter (honey)
Dinner	**Grilled Bison Steak** 4 oz bison steak Broccoli Spinach salad with 1 oz goat cheese	**Baked Wild Salmon** 3 oz salmon, brushed with olive oil and baked, skin side down, for about 10 minutes at 425°F Steamed artichoke Mixed green salad with 1 Tbsp vinaigrette (honey, nutmeg, and cinnamon) ½ cup quinoa	**Turkey Burger** 4 oz ground turkey formed into a burger patty and served on whole-wheat English muffin (pepper, fresh herbs, dried spices, ketchup, Worcestershire sauce) 1 slice reduced-fat cheese Beet chips Arugula and tomato salad with 2 tsp vinaigrette	**Pork Tenderloin** 4 oz pork tenderloin seasoned with salt and pepper and roasted at 350°F for 15 minutes (paprika or Moroccan spice mix) Steamed green beans Spinach salad with sliced cherry tomatoes and red onions

(A serving of almonds should fit in the cupped palm of your hand.)

week 6

	MONDAY	TUESDAY	WEDNESDAY
Breakfast	**Egg White Wrap** 3 scrambled egg whites topped with 1 oz reduced-fat Cheddar cheese wrapped in small whole-wheat tortilla Small fat-free latte	**PB Waffle** 1 whole-grain frozen waffle spread with 2 tsp natural peanut butter 1 cup fat-free milk 1 cup diced papaya	**Muesli** ⅓ cup rolled oats, 1 Tbsp wheat germ, 5 chopped almonds, and 3 chopped dried apricots served over ¾ cup fat-free plain yogurt
Snack	15 tamari almonds	8 pecan halves 2 dried figs	1 oz herbed goat cheese spread onto endive
Lunch	**Hearty Soup** 1 cup black bean soup Mixed green salad with 2 tsp vinaigrette and 2 high-fiber crackers (guacamole)	**Mediterranean Platter** 2 high-fiber crackers, 6 large olives, 4 Tbsp hummus, and sliced cucumber and red and yellow bell peppers	**Hummus Sandwich** ½ whole-wheat pita, 2 Tbsp hummus, cucumber, tomato, alfalfa sprouts, baby spinach, and 4 olives
Post-Workout Snack	1 cup fat-free chocolate milk 8 almonds	¾ cup nonfat plain Greek yogurt (honey) 3 Tbsp wheat germ	**Sweet-Potato Chips** 1 small sweet potato, thinly sliced and placed on baking sheet coated with cooking spray; sprinkle with sea salt and bake at 375°F for 25 minutes, or until crispy
Dinner	**Grilled Steak** 4 oz beef tenderloin Steamed cauliflower, mashed with 2 Tbsp Parmesan cheese (chicken broth to help soften) Steamed green beans	**Asian Stir Fry** 4 oz firm tofu, drained and cubed, sautéed with bok choy in 2 tsp olive oil and topped with 1 Tbsp sesame seeds Mixed green salad with 1 Tbsp vinaigrette	**Grilled Chicken** 4 oz boneless, skinless chicken breast Steamed asparagus Mixed green salad with 2 tsp vinaigrette

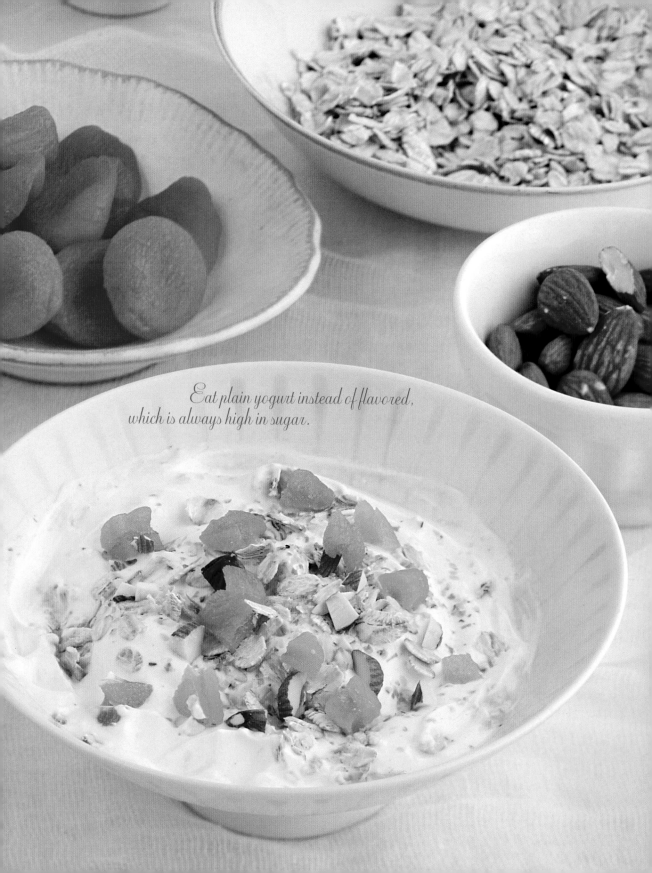

Eat plain yogurt instead of flavored, which is always high in sugar.

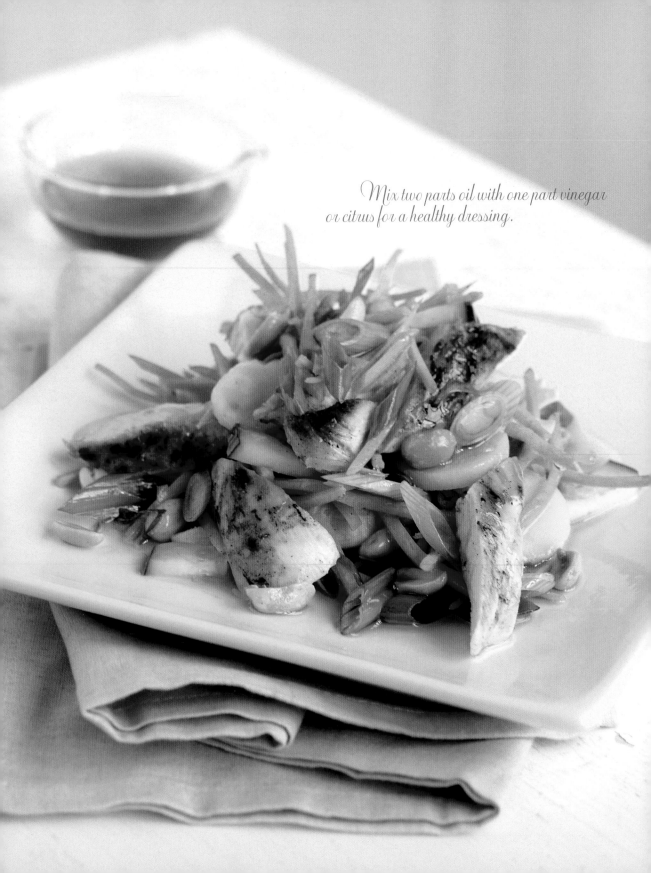

Mix two parts oil with one part vinegar or citrus for a healthy dressing.

How much are you *actually* eating?

A 4-ounce serving of chicken is about the same size as the palm of a woman's hand.

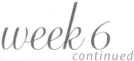

week 6
continued

	THURSDAY	FRIDAY	SATURDAY	SUNDAY
Breakfast	**Broiled Grapefruit** ½ grapefruit sprinkled with cinnamon and broiled until top is bubbly, and served with 1 slice whole-wheat toast spread with 2 tsp almond butter 1 cup fat-free milk	**Hearty Cereal** ¾ oat bran flakes with 1 cup fat-free milk, 1 Tbsp chopped macadamia nuts, and 1 cup raspberries	**Salmon Sandwich** 1 toasted whole-wheat English muffin, spread with ½ cup whipped cottage cheese, and topped with 2 oz smoked salmon	**Apple Cinnamon Oatmeal** 1 packet plain instant oatmeal prepared with fat-free milk, topped with 7 chopped walnut halves and ½ of a chopped apple (cinnamon)
Snack	1 Tbsp guacamole 6 jicama slices or carrot sticks	1 cup steamed edamame (pepper)	1 hard-boiled egg	1 oz 50 percent reduced-fat Cheddar cheese Sliced red and yellow bell peppers
Lunch	**Veggie Burger** 1 veggie burger topped with ½ of a sliced avocado on toasted English muffin (salsa) Mixed green salad (lemon juice and vinegar)	**Asian Chicken Salad** 4 oz grilled chicken, sliced water chestnuts, carrots, scallions, and cucumber with 2 tsp sesame oil and brown rice vinegar	**Grilled Salmon Salad** 4 oz grilled salmon over romaine lettuce with 1 oz reduced-fat feta cheese, cherry tomatoes, and 1 Tbsp vinaigrette	**"Chicken Wing" Salad** 4 oz grilled chicken breast (hot sauce) over romaine lettuce, carrots, celery, and 1 Tbsp crumbled blue cheese
Post-Workout Snack	100-calorie pack microwave popcorn, sprinkled with 3 Tbsp Parmesan cheese	2 Tbsp hummus on small whole-wheat wrap with sliced tomato	**Tart Shake** 1 cup nonfat plain Greek yogurt, 1 cup ice, ½ cup frozen unsweetened cherries, and 1 Tbsp flaxseed (2 mint leaves)	1 apple 2 tsp peanut butter
Dinner	**Pan-Cooked Tilapia** 4 oz tilapia cooked 2 to 3 minutes per side (Spanish spice mix and served with Mango salsa) Roasted brussels sprouts Mixed green salad with 2 tsp vinaigrette Small baked sweet potato	**Spaghetti Squash** 1 spaghetti squash, halved and seeds removed; microwave (cut side up, covered with plastic wrap) for 12 minutes and scrape out flesh with a fork. Mix with marinara sauce, 2 Tbsp Parmesan cheese, and 3 small turkey meatballs.	**Pork Tenderloin** 4 oz pork tenderloin seasoned with salt and pepper and roasted at 350°F for 15 minutes (paprika or Moroccan spice mix) Steamed artichoke Mixed green salad with 1 Tbsp vinaigrette	**Shrimp and Linguine** 5 medium shrimp (sautéed, baked, or grilled), tossed with ½ cup whole-wheat pasta (any style), and 2 tsp olive oil Steamed broccoli (2 Tbsp grated Parmesan cheese)

the look better naked

total-body exercise plan

Boost your metabolism,
reshape your muscles, and reveal
a sexier shape in just 6 weeks

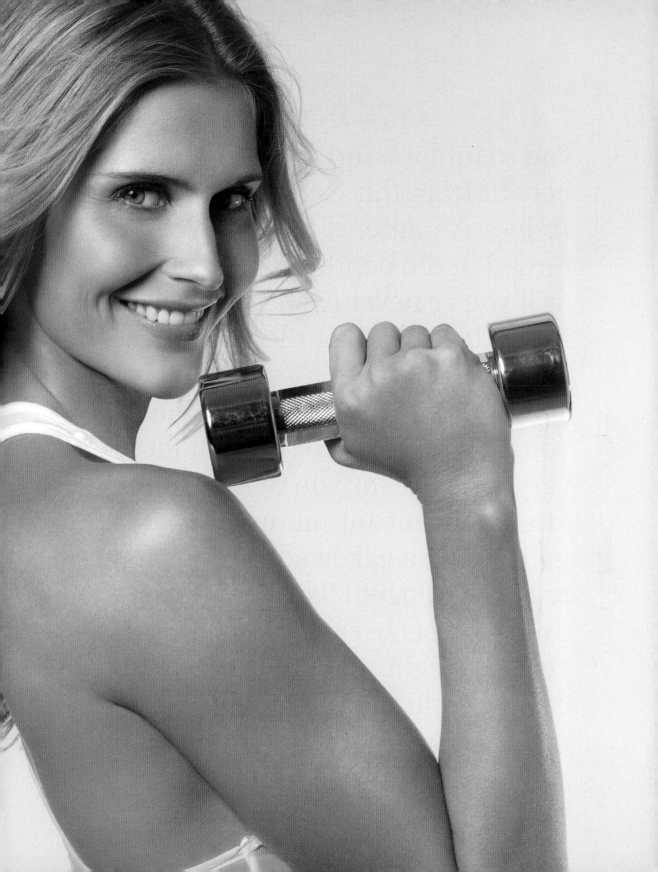

Before I get into the details, I want you to understand that *anybody* can benefit from this exercise program. It doesn't matter if your gym card is buried in the depths of your purse, or if you've never exercised at all. No matter what your level of fitness, you're going to get results you can see.

But I'm not going to lie. Whether you're stepping into the gym for the very first time or you're returning after a significant hiatus, it's not going to be a cakewalk: You're going to be challenged! That said, the program has been designed so that you can begin at a point that's comfortable for you, and progress to more and more difficult moves at a safe and gratifying rate.

The Look Better Naked workout, designed by *Women's Health* contributor Rachel Cosgrove, requires your dedication for at least 6 weeks in order to achieve the desired results. In the grand scheme of things, that's a blip on the radar screen, considering that you'll score a hot, healthier body. After those first 6 weeks, you can change up your workouts to include a mini-routine targeted to a specific trouble spot—namely, your abs, legs and butt, arms and shoulders, or breasts. Here's what you're committing to:

Your weekly schedule will include four workouts. Two will be 24-minute metabolic workouts in the form of interval training—quick bursts of high-intensity exercise followed by brief periods of rest—that you can do anywhere you want, and two will be full-body strength-training workouts. For these you can opt for the at-home equipment listed on page 5, but I recommend going to a gym. (Check out "How to Buy a Gym Membership" on page 100 to make sure you're getting the best deal possible.)

After the first 3 weeks you're going to progress to a new phase to keep boredom at bay and to ensure that your physique keeps improving. Now, I recognize that you may see promising signs of advancement well before you reach the finish line and that you'll be tempted to skip ahead. Don't let those early gains sidetrack you. I want you to follow the program in its entirety and exactly as it's written. LBN isn't about cheating your way into a better-looking body. It's about earning one.

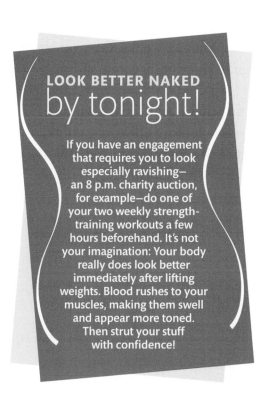

LOOK BETTER NAKED
by tonight!

If you have an engagement that requires you to look especially ravishing—an 8 p.m. charity auction, for example—do one of your two weekly strength-training workouts a few hours beforehand. It's not your imagination: Your body really does look better immediately after lifting weights. Blood rushes to your muscles, making them swell and appear more toned. Then strut your stuff with confidence!

The Science Behind Look Better Naked

For the purposes of this program, your metabolic workouts will replace cardiovascular training. These twice-a-week workouts will set the stage for visible results by torching flab. Why interval training instead of old-fashioned running? Research has shown that a conventional aerobic workout, such as jogging on a treadmill, is less effective for shedding fat. In a particularly noteworthy study published in the *International Journal of Sport Nutrition and Exercise Metabolism*, researchers tracked 91 women who completed 45 minutes of steady-state aerobic exercise at 78 percent of their maximum heart rate 5 days a week. Yet, after 12 weeks, the women in the study experienced absolutely *no change* in their body composition compared to dieting alone.

The benefits of interval training, on the other hand, have been well documented by researchers, who tout it as a much more effective method of boosting metabolism and shedding body fat. A 2008 study published in the *International Journal of Obesity* revealed that women who did 20 minutes of interval training just 3 days a week lost an average of 5.5 pounds over 15 weeks. (Two of the women even dropped 18 pounds!) Meanwhile the other group of women in the study, who performed 40 minutes of steady-state aerobics 3 days a week, *gained* a pound during the same period. "If you want to look better naked, do intervals—they'll trump those long, boring slogs on a treadmill or stair stepper every single time," says Cosgrove.

Workout designed by **Rachel Cosgrove**, a *Women's Health* advisor; co-owner of Results Fitness, based in Santa Clarita, California; and author of *The Female Body Breakthrough* (thefemalebodybreakthrough.com).

The goal of the two strength workouts, on the other hand, is to build lean body mass—that is, to strengthen your skeletal muscles. They're the ones that attach to your bones via tendons, and that you use to suck in your stomach or carry heavy shopping bags to your car; in other

Interval training is a fun, high-intensity way to shed body fat, and it will always trump long, boring slogs on a treadmill or stair stepper.

words, the ones that you're most aware of as you go about your day. (The two other types of muscle in your body facilitate the movement of internal organs, such as your heart and esophagus.) Skeletal muscles make up 30 to 40 percent of your body mass and are largely voluntary, meaning *you* control their movement—except the occasional involuntary blip when someone scares the heck out of you.

Here's a quick primer on how strength training works. Imagine a handful of dry spaghetti. Each strand represents a muscle fiber. These fibers are bundled together—larger muscles, such as your quads, can pack up to 150 in one bunch—and huddle with other bundles to make up the entire muscle. This is what skeletal muscle looks like.

The number of muscle fibers you have was determined by the time you hit high school. "The number may increase early in life, but it becomes set at puberty," says C. David Geier Jr., MD, director of sports medicine at the Medical University of South Carolina. What you *can* control is how big the fibers get, which determines how tight and strong you look.

Increasing the size of a muscle fiber is a matter of injury and recovery. When you cut your finger, your body heals, but it often overcompensates by leaving a scab. Something similar happens with your muscles. Every time that you lift a barbell, beach bag, or baby, the action can cause microscopic tears in the muscle fibers. As a result, your muscles send a signal to nearby cells to come to the rescue. These cells trigger the formation of proteins at the site of the muscle tears, the body then repairs and reinforces the fibers, and that strengthens the muscle.

But fear not—regular strength training won't turn you into the Incredible Hulkette. First and foremost, there's a biological explanation for this: A woman's body produces 20 to 30 percent less testosterone than a man's. We gain strength and tone; they gain strength and bulk. Plus, these weight workouts will focus on an innovative technique that the *Women's Health* fitness editors and I have dubbed "featherweight strength training." It's a more approachable take on weightlifting — one that will not only boost your metabolism, but will also help you sculpt muscle definition in your arms, butt, legs, and abs, which is vitally important to achieving a sexier body.

The Basic LBN Framework

One of the best aspects of this program is its succinctness: You have four workouts to complete each week, yet you'll be in the gym for a total of less than 3 hours. It's also intended to be incredibly flexible. If you do your first strength workout and plan to do your metabolic workout the next morning but something comes up—maybe you feel too sore or your sister calls with a crisis—that's fine. Simply get it done the next day. Plus you don't have to stick to any set routine. Just find a way to finish two strength-training workouts and two metabolic workouts each week. The only rule: Avoid doing the program's workouts 3 days in a row. Your body needs recovery time in order to get tighter and leaner. For example, your week might look like one of the following options, but there are plenty of other combinations you can put together on your own:

pick a training plan
(or make your own!)

MONDAY	TUESDAY	WEDNESDAY	THURSDAY	FRIDAY	SATURDAY	SUNDAY
Strength Workout A	Metabolic Workout	OFF	Strength Workout B	Metabolic Workout	OFF	Do-Anything Day (Optional)
Metabolic Workout	OFF	Strength Workout A	Metabolic Workout	Do-Anything Day (Optional)	OFF	Strength Workout B
OFF	Strength Workout A	Do-Anything Day (Optional)	OFF	Metabolic Workout	Strength Workout B	Metabolic Workout
OFF	Metabolic Workout	Strength Workout A	OFF	Do-Anything Day (Optional)	Strength Workout B	Metabolic Workout
OFF	Strength Workout A	Metabolic Workout	Do-Anything Day (Optional)	OFF	Metabolic Workout	Strength Workout B
OFF	Strength Workout A	Metabolic Workout	OFF	Metabolic Workout	Strength Workout B	Do-Anything Day (Optional)
Strength Workout A	OFF	Strength Workout B	Metabolic Workout	OFF	Metabolic Workout	Do-Anything Day (Optional)

Your Optional Do-Anything Day

Think of this as an "active recovery day"—an opportunity to enjoy any activity you want. Catch a yoga, dance, or Pilates class; play tennis; ride your bike; go for an easy jog; or just take a walk—anything you want to do. The key is that it cannot interfere with your recovery and take away from your four LBN workouts. If you're feeling spent, don't push yourself. Just use the day to chill.

Stay local. Consider only those gyms within a 15-minute drive of where you live or work. Joining one that's farther away will dramatically reduce your chances of staying committed to your exercise program. Once you've narrowed the field by distance and pinpointed a few gyms that seem to meet your needs, follow these tips to ensure a good fit—and the best possible deal.

HOW TO BUY A GYM MEMBERSHIP

Be wary of perks. If you don't plan to use more than half of a club's services, find yourself another club. Perks inflate membership fees. Many gyms charge extra for classes and facilities. Some even require an additional fee to rent a locker.

Check credentials. A health club is only as good as its instructors. The National Commission for Certifying Agencies accredits more than 190 certifying programs, the most common of which are abbreviated as NASM, ACE, NSCA, CI-CPT, ACSM, NESTA, NETA, NFPT, and NCSF. If you see any of these acronyms on trainers' certificates or after their names, you'll be in good hands.

Try before you buy.
Get a trial membership and go to the gym at the time you'd normally work out to get a sense of how crowded it will be when you're most likely to be there. Make sure the equipment doesn't squeak and the weights are stacked properly—two signs that the gym is managed effectively.

Go low. Gym memberships are negotiable, and managers can approve any price to seal the deal as long as they don't go lower than a predetermined rate. Don't think they'll bargain? In a survey taken at the beginning of 2009 by the American Council on Fitness, 48 percent of fitness professionals believed that the number of gym memberships would decrease by year's end. Gain the upper hand by researching the membership fees, amenities, and services offered by a gym's competitors, and don't be afraid to walk away from the table. Many clubs would rather waive your activation fee, give you a free month, or offer you extra services than lose your business.

The Gym Calculator

Should you switch plans?

A. What do you currently pay per month? _____

B. What does your gym charge for a single visit? _____

C. How often do you plan to visit the gym in the next month? _____

D. Divide C by 2: _____

If
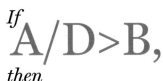
$$A/D > B,$$
then
choose the pay-as-you-go plan. If not, consider a flat-rate annual plan.

Pay per visit. If you're serious about tightening your belt—financially as well as physically—consider paying as you go. "Gym users with monthly memberships pay 70 percent more than those on pay-as-you-go plans based on actual usage," says Stefano Della Vigna, PhD, an assistant professor of economics at the University of California at Berkeley who studied 7,752 gym users over 3 years. "When we join a gym, we confuse what we'd like to do in the future with what we will actually do." Plus, monthly contracts are automatically renewed, and an average of 2 months usually elapses between a user's final visit and their actual cancellation, leading to a greater waste of money, says Della Vigna. Use the gym calculator on the left to determine whether you should opt for this below-the-radar approach.

the
featherweight
strength
workout

➡ Entering a weight room can be intimidating. Don't worry: Once you master the moves, you'll feel right at home—and when you see how dramatically (and quickly!) your body transforms, you'll be too psyched to feel uncomfortable. While you're here, I want you to use weights that you can safely handle and that will allow you to maintain your form and tempo for each exercise and complete the designated number of repetitions. If you're not in your best physical condition at the start of the program, use very light weights, say, 2-, 3-, or 5-pounders—or even

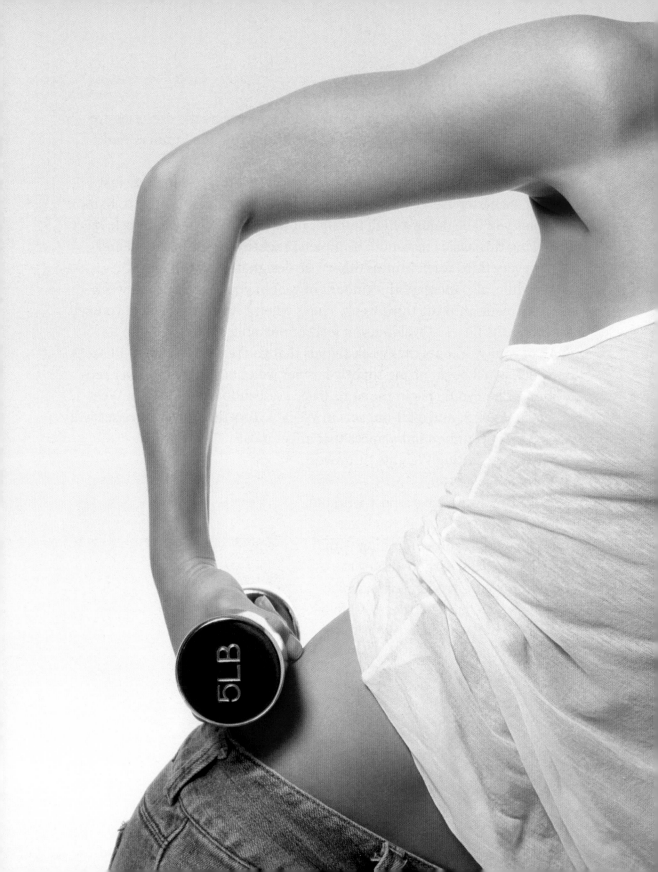

just your own body weight. The terms I use to describe the exercises are pretty basic, but if you happen to see something you don't understand, refer to "How to Use This Workout."

During the first week of this program, I want you to complete just 1 set of each exercise. It will be enough stimulation for your body to handle, plus you'll be doing a high number of repetitions. The next week, start following this basic crescendo: Complete 2 sets every second week and 3 sets every third week (unless otherwise designated, as in Phase 1). Meanwhile, also increase the amount of weight you're lifting each week by 10 percent until the third week. That's when I want you to push yourself by lifting the heaviest weights you feel comfortable using. Doing so for both of your workouts that week signals that you're ready to begin Phase 2, in which you'll begin lifting slightly heavier weights and doing fewer repetitions. Then you'll begin the same basic crescendo again: 1 set in Week 1, 2 sets in Week 2, and 3 all-out sets in Week 3. Together these exercises will help correct common imbalances that affect most women (see "Lifting Weights Improves Posture" on page 139).

Lastly, always have a post-workout snack or drink as soon as you leave the gym—preferably something with both protein and carbohydrates to replenish your glycogen levels, which will be depleted after strength training. You'll find specific postworkout snacks in Chapter 3.

The 1-Hour Rule

On featherweight strength-training days, I want you in and out of the gym in less than an hour—including your warmup. If your workout is taking you longer than an hour, monitor your rest periods more closely. People frequently take longer breathers than they need to. Sixty seconds is the longest break you should take.

How to Use This Workout

Labels: In the descriptions of these workouts, when you see an exercise preceded by the same number and different letters, these are intended to be completed as a pair (Phase 1) or a triad (Phase 2). Alternate between them before moving on to the next exercises. If you see 1A and 1B, and 2A and 2B, for example, do 1 set of 1A and rest, followed by 1 set of 1B, and rest again. Complete all your sets of that pair of exercises and then move to 2A and 2B.

Reps: Short for repetitions, this refers to how many times you'll repeat a given exercise in a set.

Rest: This is how long you recover, in seconds, before starting the next exercise. Stick to your rest periods and don't get sidetracked chatting with someone or drinking water like a camel.

Sets: This term refers to how many groups of repetitions of an exercise you will do in a workout. In this program you'll do 1 to 2 sets in Phase 1 and from then on you'll do up to 3 sets. Each set should last a designated period of time. If you do the reps too quickly, your set will be over much sooner than if you do them at the appropriate tempo.

Tempo: This is how fast you perform each repetition. Despite its importance, many strength-training programs neglect to mention it. This program uses a moderate tempo, which should take you about 2 seconds to lift the weight and 2 seconds to lower it—and the movement should be under control during that time. Pay close attention to maintaining that tempo, which will help you achieve the program's goals and get you out of the gym on time.

➤➤ Begin every strength workout with this warmup. As you will quickly discover, it's a much better way to get limber than jogging on a treadmill. Once you've completed these 10 exercises, which should take less than 10 minutes from start to finish, you'll be ready for a more effective workout.

the dynamic warmup

instructions: Complete the following exercises one after another without stopping, and then transition straight into the first lifting exercise. After a few weeks the routine will become second nature to you, but resist the temptation to speed through it. Concentrate on improving the range of motion for each joint, getting your limbs loose, and raising your heart rate.

exercise	reps	sets
Pivoting Deep Squat	20	1
Walking Leg Cradle	10/side	1
Walking Heel to Butt	10/side	1
Lateral Jump	20	1
Walking Inverted Hamstrings	10/side	1
Wide Outs	20	1
Forward and Back Single-Leg Hop	10/side	1
Lunge Walk with Rotation and Overhead Reach	10/side	1
Single-Leg Lateral Hop	10/side	1
Lateral Pushup Shuffle	5/side	1

pivoting deep squat

start

- Stand with your feet wide apart and your arms reaching overhead as high as you can.

movement

- Keeping both arms reaching toward the ceiling, squat as low as you can. Hold your torso as upright as possible.

- Straighten your legs and pivot around to face the opposite direction and perform the exact same move again to complete 1 rep.

- Repeat, alternating directions the entire time, while keeping your arms straight up overhead.

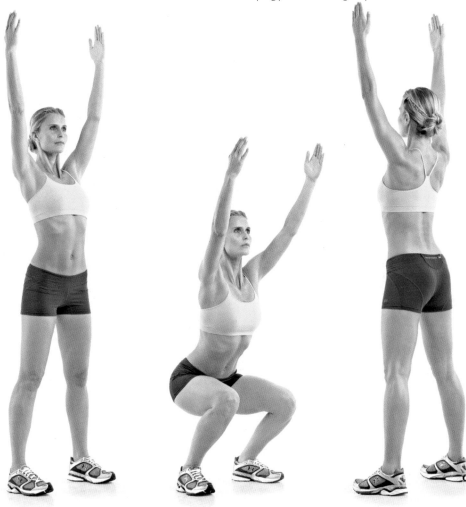

walking leg cradle

start
- Stand with your feet together.

movement
- Raise your right knee and grab it with your right hand. Then, with your left hand, grab the outside of your right ankle and pull your foot up so the foot is even with your hip. Keeping your back straight, bend your left knee and lower your butt until you feel a stretch in your right hip.

- Lower your leg after a second or so, return to the starting position, and repeat on the opposite side. Take a step each time you alternate legs.

walking heel to butt

start
- Stand with your feet shoulder-width apart and your arms at your sides.

movement
- Bend your right knee, bringing your right heel to your right butt cheek, and grab your foot with your right hand. Balancing on your left foot, keep your right knee pointed toward the floor so that you feel a stretch in your right quadriceps and hip flexor for a few seconds. Take a step as you bring your right foot to the floor and then repeat on the other side.

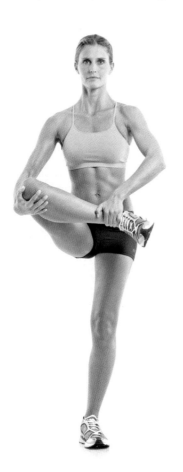 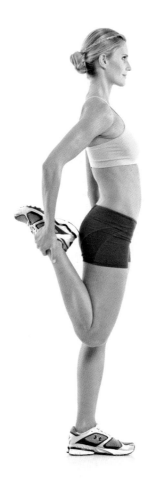

lateral jump

start

- Stand with your feet together and your knees slightly bent. Now imagine there's a line drawn on the floor about 3 inches to your right.

movement

- With both feet together, jump over the line laterally and land 3 inches to the right of the line with your feet still together. Keep your knees bent while jumping and landing.

- Immediately jump back to your starting position to complete 1 rep. Continue to repeat this motion as quickly as you can by exploding back and forth over the line. You might even want to pretend that the floor is hot to keep it interesting!

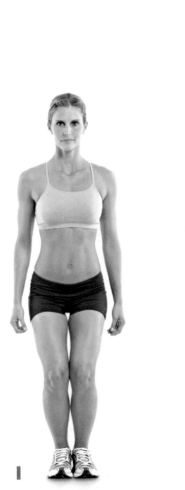
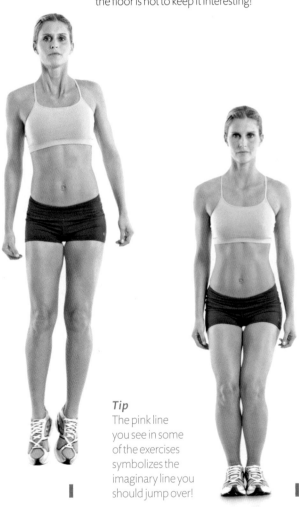

Tip
The pink line you see in some of the exercises symbolizes the imaginary line you should jump over!

walking inverted hamstring

start

- Stand with your feet shoulder-width apart.

movement

- Step forward, putting your weight on your left leg. As if you were a teeter-totter, balance on your left leg and lift your right leg straight behind you, allowing your torso to bend forward to form a straight line from your head through your right leg.

- Keep your hips square. You should feel a stretch in your left hamstring. Bring your right leg down to the starting position and repeat on the other side.

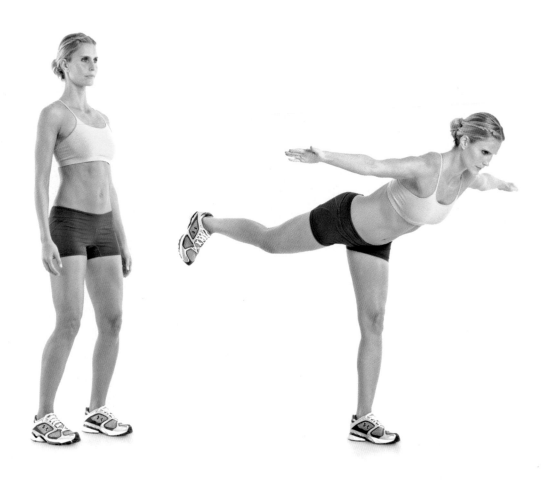

wide out

start

- Stand with your feet together and your arms straight out in front of you at shoulder height, with your palms facing each other.

movement

- Jump and spread your legs so that you land, heels first, with your feet wide apart. While you're jumping, simultaneously open your arms so that they extend straight out to your sides. Close your arms as you jump back to the starting position.

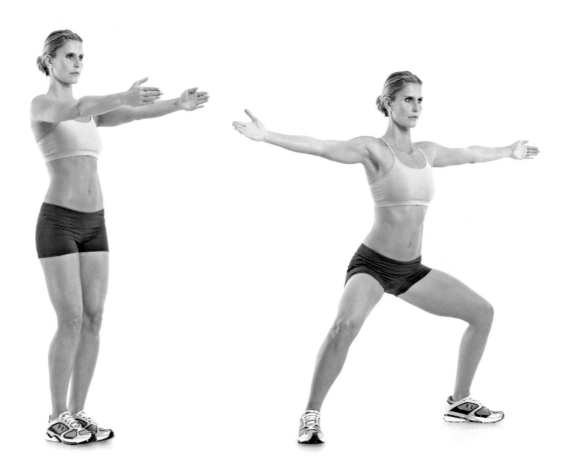

forward and back single-leg hop

start

- Stand on your right leg. Imagine there's a line drawn on the floor 3 inches in front of you.

movement

- Jump over the line with your right leg and land on your right foot 3 inches from the line.

- Then jump backward over the line to the starting position. That's 1 rep.

- Keep the jumps small and, again, pretend the floor is hot so that you do them quickly. Do all the reps on your right leg before switching to your left.

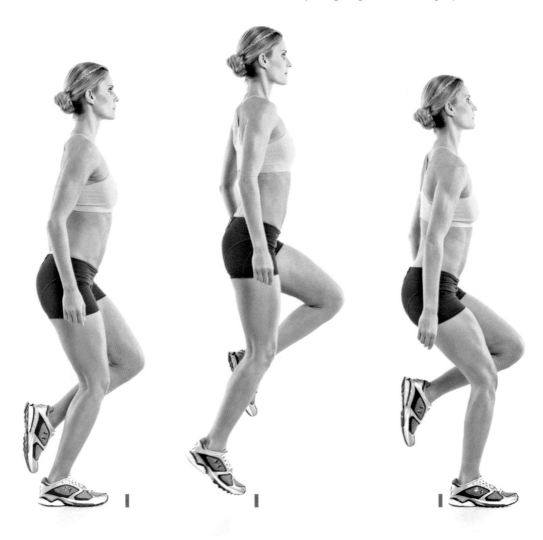

lunge walk with rotation and overhead reach

start

- Stand with your feet about shoulder-width apart and your arms at your sides.

movement

- Step forward with your right leg and lower yourself into a deep lunge.

- As you lunge, rotate your torso over the front leg and raise your arms straight up overhead.

- Bring your left leg forward to stand upright again and repeat with your left leg.

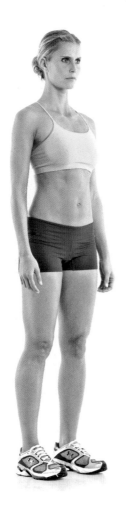

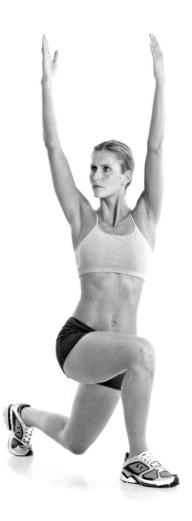

single-leg lateral hop

start

- Stand on your right leg. Imagine there's a line drawn on the floor 3 inches to your left.

movement

- Jump over the line with your right leg, land on your right foot, and then jump back over, landing on the same foot to complete 1 rep.

- Keep the jumps small and, again, pretend the floor is hot. Do all your reps with your right leg, then repeat with your left leg (starting with the imaginary line at your left side).

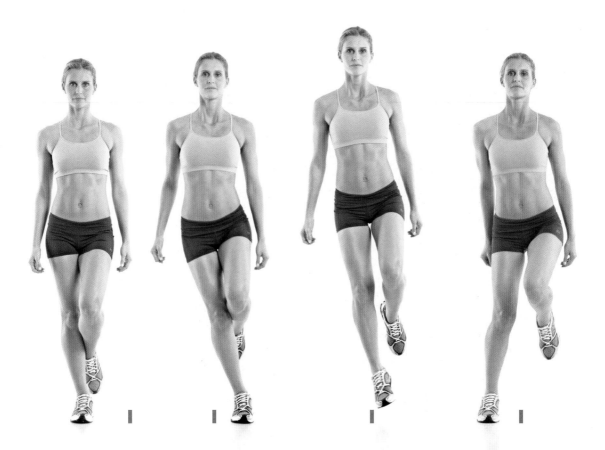

lateral pushup shuffle

start
- Get into a st andard pushup position with your hips, shoulders, and head in a straight line.

movement
- Moving laterally, position your right hand and right foot about 7 or 8 inches farther to the right and then resume the standard pushup position by moving your left hand and left foot 7 or 8 inches toward the right.

- Shuffle to the right for 5 reps, then switch and shuffle to the left for 5 reps.

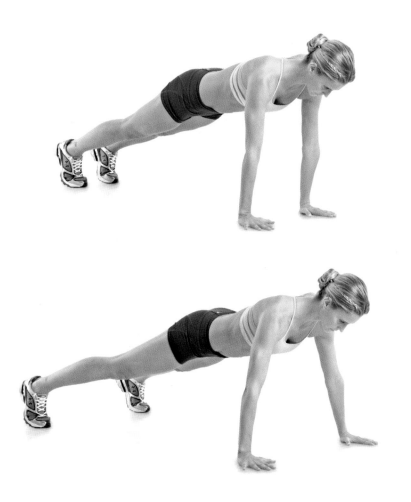

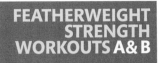

phase 1: WEEKS 1 TO 3

strength workout A

EXERCISE	SETS	REPS	TEMPO/TIME	REST
Dynamic Warmup	See page 106			
1A: Plank	1–2	1	30–60 sec	30 sec
1B: Prone Cobra	1–2	1/side	30–60 sec	60 sec
2A: Hip Extension	1–2	15	moderate	30 sec
2B: Four-Way Raise*	1–2	5/position	moderate	60 sec
3A: Stationary Lunge*	1–2	15/side	moderate	30 sec
3B: Incline Pushup	1–2	15	moderate	60 sec
4A: Three-Point Dumbbell Row*	1–2	15/side	moderate	30 sec
4B: Single-Leg, Single-Arm Reach	1–2	15/side	moderate	60 sec

strength workout B

EXERCISE	SETS	REPS	TEMPO/TIME	REST
Dynamic Warmup	See page 106			
1A: Side Plank	1–2	1/side	15-30 sec/side	30 sec
1B: Plank with Alternate Arm and Leg Reach	1–2	10/side	moderate	60 sec
2A: Supine Hip Extension on Swiss Ball	1–2	15	moderate	30 sec
2B: Wood Chop*	1–2	15/side	moderate	60 sec
3A: Stepup*	1–2	15/side	moderate	30 sec
3B: Standing Alternating Lateral Raise*	1–2	15/side	moderate	60 sec
4A: Overhead Squat*	1–2	15	moderate	30 sec
4B: Close-Grip Pulldown*	1–2	15	moderate	60 sec

*Add weight as you progress in the program

1A
plank

Position

• Lie belly-down on the floor. Rise onto your forearms and your toes, keeping your back in a straight line. Tighten your abdominals to keep yourself stable. This is a static exercise—there's no movement—so you'll simply hold this position for the designated time without compromising your form.

Don't Cut That Corner!

Three weeks is the minimum you'll need for each phase of the program. And just because this part is called "Phase 1" doesn't mean it's a beginner's workout. Even if you're in great shape you will benefit from these 3 weeks. Use the progressions and regressions in the exercise descriptions to complement your fitness level.

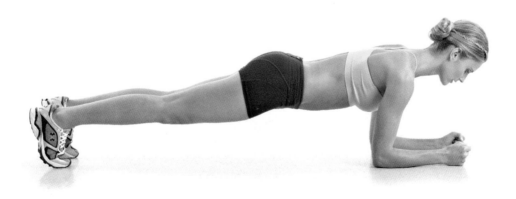

1B
prone cobra

start

- Lie facedown on a mat or carpeted floor and rest your arms at your sides, palms down.

movement

- Contract the muscles in your glutes and lower back so that your upper torso and legs come off the floor.

- At the same time, rotate your arms externally so that your thumbs end up pointed toward the ceiling. Keep a neutral neck alignment. Hold this position. If you cannot hold for the desired time, regress the exercise by doing multiple reps of a 5- to 10-second hold.

Tip
As you get stronger, try to balance your torso on a Swiss ball instead.

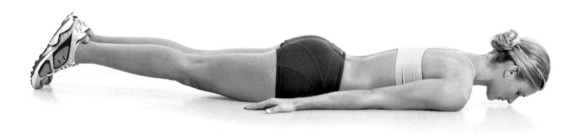

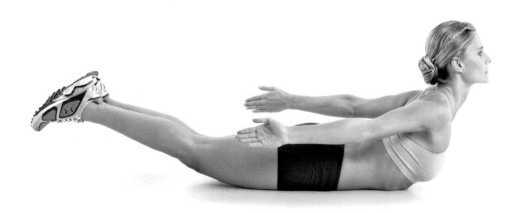

hip extension

start

• Lie on your back. Bend your knees so your feet are flat on the floor. Place your arms at your sides, palms up.

movement

• Tighten your core. Now squeeze your glutes to lift your hips off the floor and toward the ceiling until your body forms a straight line from your shoulders to your knees. Lower yourself to the starting position.

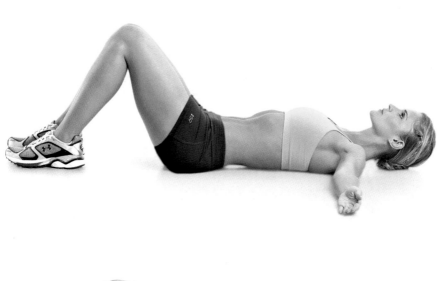

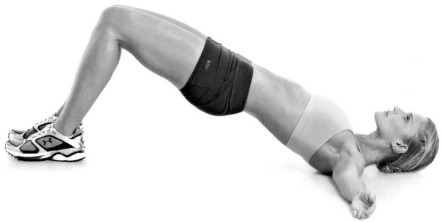

2B
four-way raise

start

• For this exercise you'll position your upper body to form four letters: Y, T, W, and I (the exercise is often called "YTWI" for this reason). Start in a squat. Lean forward so your torso is at a 45-degree angle. Lift your arms over your head to form a "Y."

movement

• Keeping your arms straight in the "Y" position, move them up and down five times, pulling your shoulder blades toward each other as you do so; the movement should be very small, to keep your upper back muscles contracted.

• Then take your arms straight out to the sides, forming a "T," with your thumbs pointing toward the ceiling. Perform the same movement in this position five times.

• Then bend your arms at the elbow, forming a "W" shape, as if you are flapping your wings. Raise and lower your arms five times, again pulling your shoulder blades toward each other. Finally, form your body into an "I" by extending your arms straight in front of you. Raise your arms as far as you can. Lower them and repeat for a total of 5 repetitions.

Tip
If standing proves too difficult, lie facedown on a bench.

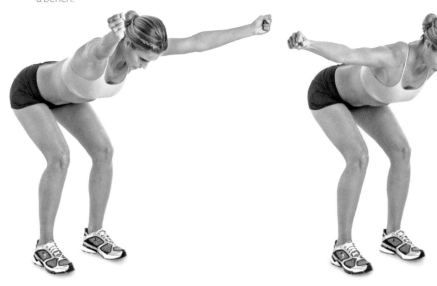

movement *(continued)*

- Then bend your arms at the elbow, forming a "W" shape, as if you are flapping your wings. Raise and lower your arms five times, again pulling your shoulder blades toward each other.

- Finally, form your body into an "I" by extending your arms straight in front of you. Raise your arms as far as you can. Lower them and repeat for a total of 5 repetitions.

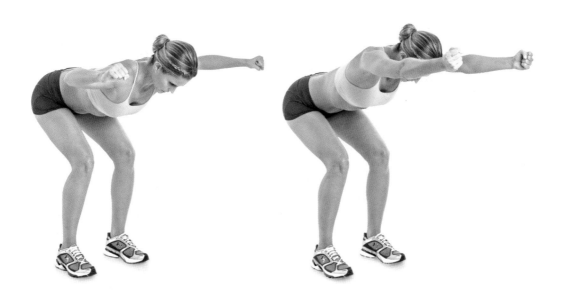

stationary lunge

start

- Begin with one foot about 2 or 3 feet in front of the other and space them shoulder-width apart. Stand tall with your arms at your sides. Hold dumbbells in both hands.

movement

- Slowly lower yourself into a lunge by dropping your rear knee down until it almost touches the floor. Keep your right knee tracking over your toes. When your right thigh is just past parallel with the floor, pause, and then drive the heel of your right foot into the floor and return to the starting position. That's 1 rep.

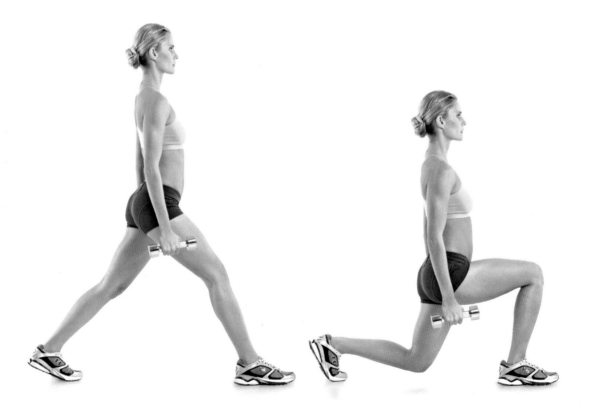

3B
incline pushup

start

- Get into the pushup position with your hands on a step or bench. (If you are strong enough to do real pushups on the floor, do so—otherwise the higher the incline the easier this will be.) Your spine should be in a straight line, with your head, upper back, and tailbone in alignment.

movement

- Bend your elbows and lower your entire body toward the floor, keeping your abdominals tight, until your shoulders are just below your elbows. Return to the start position, again keeping your body in a straight line. If you cannot get the full range of motion without letting your back arch or sticking your hips out, increase the incline.

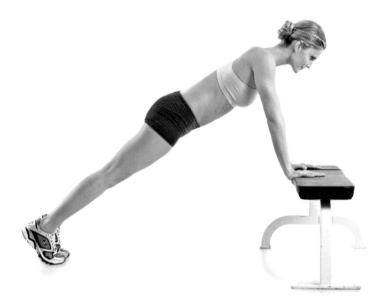

Tip
Lower the height of the incline as you progress in the program.

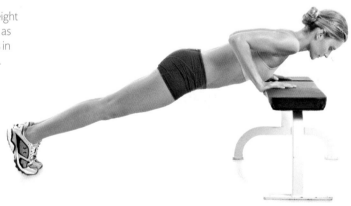

4A
three-point dumbbell row

start
- Bend forward and place your left hand on a bench. Your feet should be directly under your hips, shoulder-width apart, and your back should be flat, with your head, spine, and tailbone in a straight line. Hold a dumbbell in your right hand, keeping your right arm straight and pointed toward the floor.

movement
- Row the dumbbell up to your body by squeezing your shoulder blade back. Maintain a neutral spine. Lower the dumbbell and repeat. Do not shrug your shoulder; the movement should all be from your back. Complete all the repetitions with your right arm before repeating with your left arm.

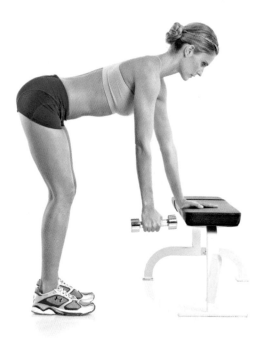
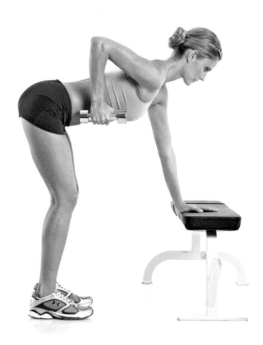

4B

single-leg, single-arm reach

start

- Stand with a neutral spine. Put all of your weight on your left leg. Raise your right foot slightly. Extend your right arm directly in front of you at shoulder height.

movement

- Push your hips back a few inches, keeping your back straight. Bend at the waist and reach for the ground with your right hand.

- As you descend, raise your right leg behind your body. You'll feel a stretch in your left hamstring.

- Go as low as you can while maintaining a neutral spine. Pause at the bottom and then slowly return to the starting postion. Do all your reps and then repeat for the opposite side of your body.

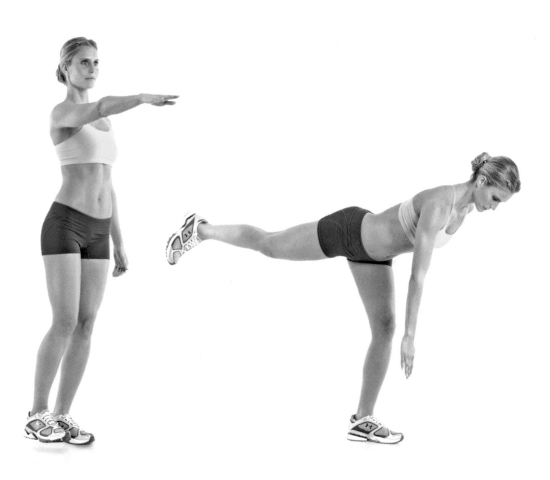

phase 1: WEEKS 1 TO 3

1A
side plank

Position

- Lie on your left side with your elbow underneath your shoulder. Your body should be in a straight line with your legs stacked one on top of the other. Balancing on your forearm and your foot, raise your hips as high as you can. Keep your core tight. This is a static exercise, so hold this position for the specified period of time, rest, and then switch sides.

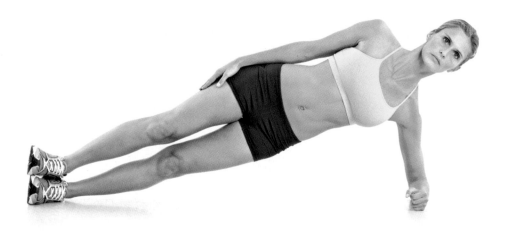

1B
plank with alternate arm and leg reach

start
- Get into the pushup position. Draw your stomach in tight, which will recruit your abdominals to keep your torso stable during the exercise.

movement
- Simultaneously lift your left arm and right leg, extending and straightening both until they're level with your torso. Return to the starting position and repeat with your right arm and left leg.

Tip
An easier version of this exercise is called bird dog. Begin in a kneeling position with your thighs perpendicular to the floor and knees shoulder-width apart, but keep your left knee planted when you raise your left arm, and vice versa.

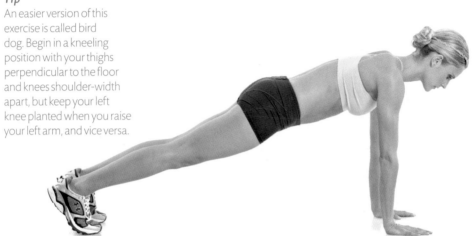

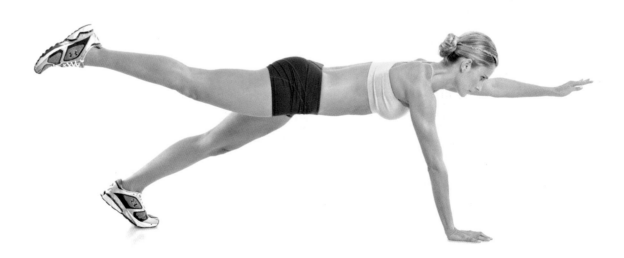

2A

supine hip extension on swiss ball

start
• Lie on your back with the back of your lower legs straight and propped on a Swiss ball. Your arms should extend to your sides, palms facing up.

movement
• Squeeze your glutes, lifting your hips off the floor and toward the ceiling. Keep your legs straight and your core tight. Raise your hips until your body forms a straight line from your shoulders through your hips and knees to your ankles. Lower yourself to the starting position.

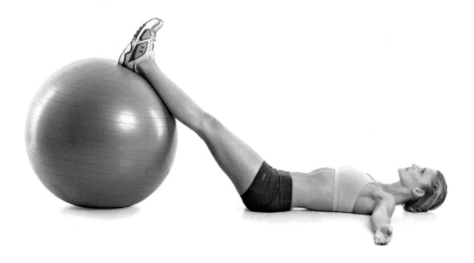

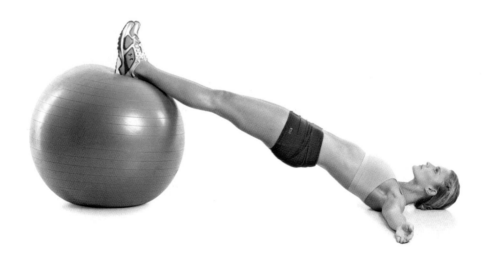

2B
wood chop

start
- Stand with a high pulley machine at your right side. Hold onto the handle with both hands and straighten your arms.

movement
- Keeping your arms straight and keeping your eyes on your hands, pull the handle straight across your body and downward in a diagonal motion, until it's outside your left knee. Return to the starting position under control and complete all the repetitions in this position before switching positions to repeat on the other side.

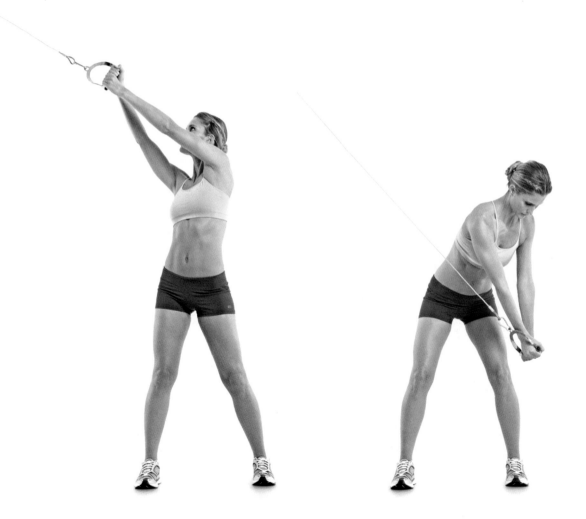

3A

stepup

start

• Stand facing a low step, holding a dumbbell in each hand. Place your left foot on the step.

movement

• Push through your left foot and lift your body up. Your right foot will leave the floor, but do not allow it to touch the step. Lower yourself to the ground under control, pause briefly, and repeat. Be sure to use only your left leg; do not bounce and push off your right. Complete all reps with your left leg before repeating with your right.

Tip

For an added challenge, increase the height of the step—eventually you'll want to use a bench. Then add load in the form of dumbbells.

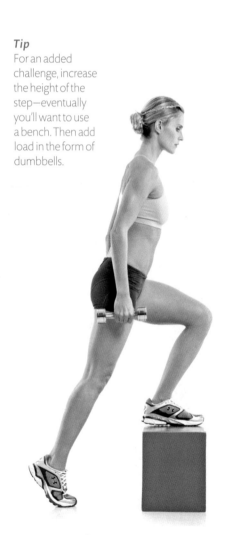

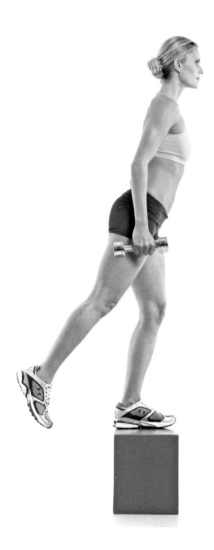

3B
standing alternating lateral raise

start
• Stand with your feet shoulder-width apart and hold a dumbbell in each hand.

movement
• Brace your abs and lift one arm straight out to the side until your hand is at shoulder height. Hold this position for a moment and then lower the weight under control. Alternate arms.

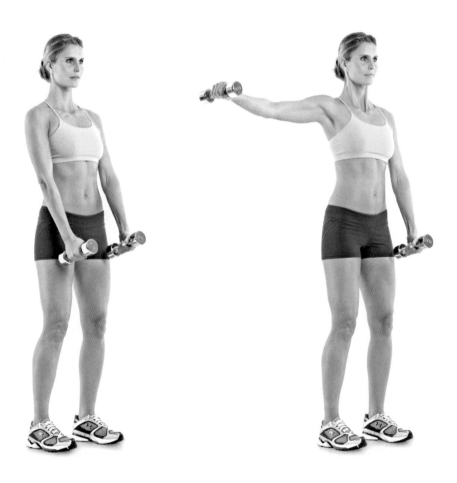

4A
overhead squat

start

- Set a bar in a squat rack above your head height. (Until your strength increases, you can use a 10- to 20-pound body bar or even a towel.) Grasp the bar with a wide overhand grip, brace your abdominals, and extend your arms overhead. Your arms should be in line with your ears.

movement

- From this position, with the bar overhead, bend at the knees and hips and lower yourself into a full squat.

- As you squat, maintain a tall posture, do not let your back round, and keep your knees aligned with your toes: Do not let them collapse inward. Keep the bar in the overhead position with your arms straight and locked during the entire movement.

- Once your thighs are just past parallel to the floor, drive upward through your heels and return to the starting position.

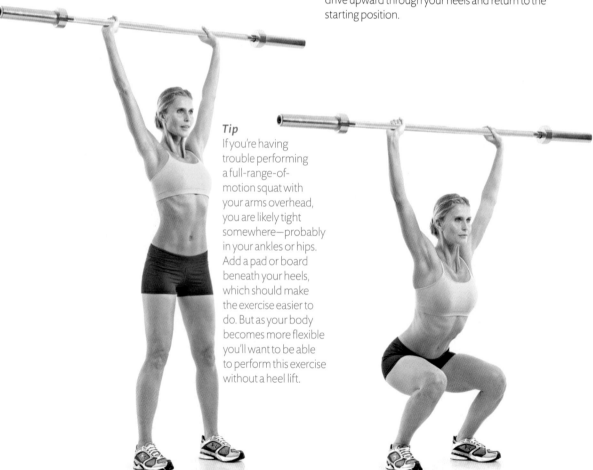

Tip

If you're having trouble performing a full-range-of-motion squat with your arms overhead, you are likely tight somewhere—probably in your ankles or hips. Add a pad or board beneath your heels, which should make the exercise easier to do. But as your body becomes more flexible you'll want to be able to perform this exercise without a heel lift.

close-grip pulldown

start

* Sit at a pulldown machine. With your hands, grab the handles or the bar at about shoulder-width apart.

movement

* Pull the bar down. (It helps if you think about pulling your chest upward.) Bring your elbows to your sides and the bar to your chest, and then slowly return to the starting position.

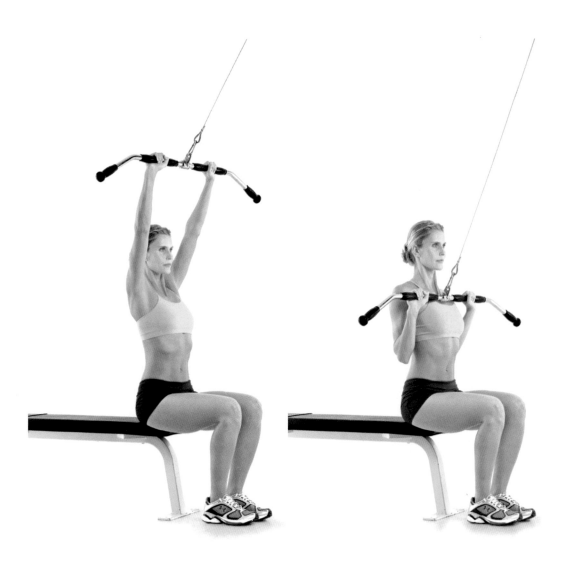

➥ Like your warmup, the interval-training workouts utilize body-weight exercises that will put you through multiple planes of motion—meaning you'll move in different directions. This will challenge your body more effectively by using multiple muscle groups. They'll also get your heart rate up, burn calories, and boost your metabolism.

Note the number of repetitions you do the first time you perform the workout. Write it down if you need to. "Each day that you repeat the routine, try to increase the number of repetitions that you complete in the same amount of time, which is also known as 'adding density,'" says Cosgrove.

the
metabolic
workout

instructions: Do each exercise as many times as you can for 30 seconds. Rest for 30 seconds and then advance to the next exercise. Complete 6 rounds total. Do not rest between rounds. These workouts should be intense and short—24 minutes is all you'll need.

phase 1: WEEKS 1 TO 3

1A Jump Squat
1B Plank to Pushup
1C Stationary Lunge
1D Jumping Rope

1A
jump squat

start
- Stand with your feet shoulder-width apart.

movement
- Keeping your torso as upright as possible, lower your body as far as you can until your thighs are at least parallel to the floor.

- Your weight should be entirely on your heels throughout this exercise, and your knees should remain over your toes when you're lowering your body.

- From the bottom position, drive yourself off the floor, exploding as high as you can into the air. Land and repeat.

Tip
For an easier version of this exercise, don't jump — just do body-weight squats instead.

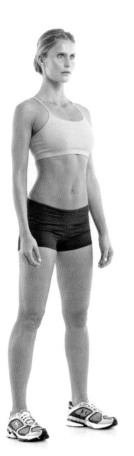
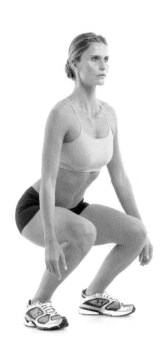
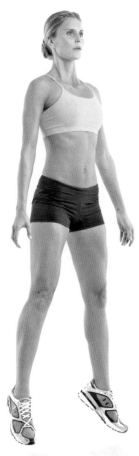

1B
plank to pushup

start

- Get into a pushup position on the floor, but instead of being on your hands, support your weight on your forearms. Your hips, shoulders, and head should form a straight line.

movement

- Keeping your core tight and your hips neutral, move your right hand into a standard pushup position and then do the same with your left hand. (At this point you'll be in the same position you would be in at the top of a pushup.)

- Return to the starting position by lowering onto your right forearm and then your left forearm. Alternate sides, rising onto your left hand next, then your right, then back to your left elbow, and then returning to the start position.

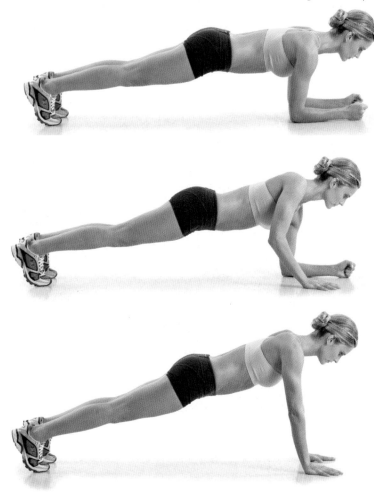

1C
stationary lunge

start
- Stand tall with your shoulders back and your feet shoulder-width apart.

movement
- Step forward into a lunge with your right leg, keeping your right knee tracking over your toes. Drive through your heel to return to the starting position. Repeat with your left leg and continue alternating legs.

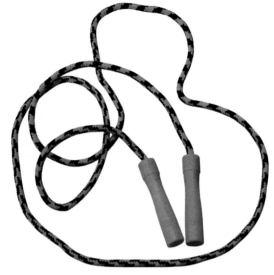

1D
jumping rope

start:
- Stand with the rope's ends in your hands. If you don't have a jump rope, pretend that you do.

movement:
- Jump rope! Vary your jumps: two feet, one foot at a time, high knees. Stay on your toes, knees bent.

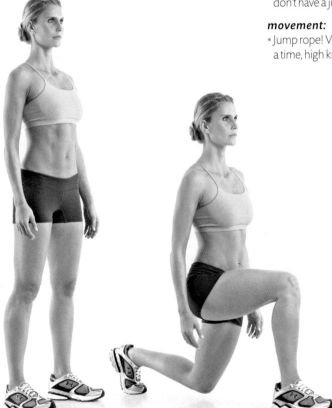

Tip
To progress this move, stay in the lunge position and drive off the ground with both legs, switching your legs in the air and landing in a lunge on the opposite leg.

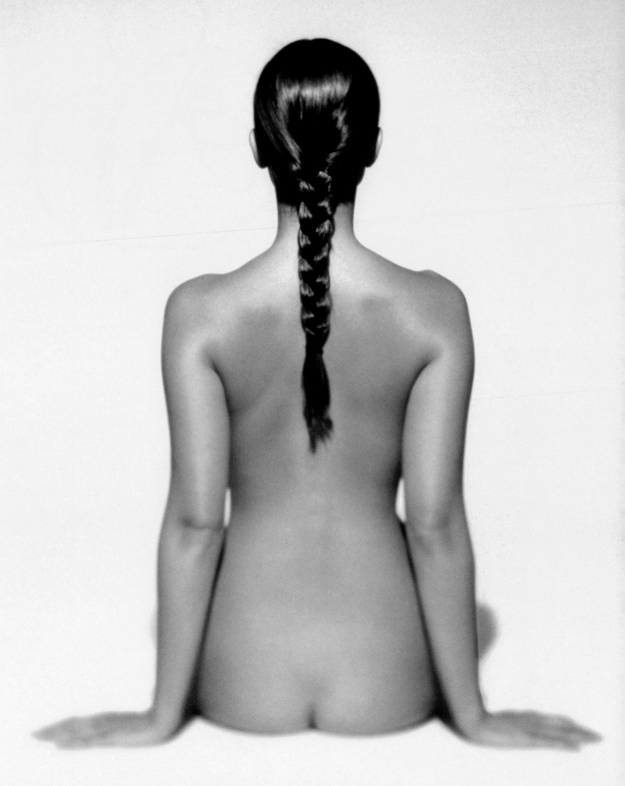

Lifting Weights Improves Posture

The featherweight strength-training program includes exercises that will improve your posture and correct some of the most common muscular imbalances among women, including:

• **Rounded, hunched shoulders.** Many of our most basic daily activities—driving a car, sitting at a desk, working at a computer, and talking on the telephone—weaken the muscles in our shoulders and necks. The LBN program is structured to restore your shoulders to their proper alignment, which will help you maintain a taller posture. And the simple act of standing taller can make you look 5 pounds lighter—without losing a single pound.

• **Tight hip flexors.** Turn perpendicular to the mirror so you can see the side of your body. Are your hips tilted forward like a duck's? Well, all that sitting also causes the tiny muscles located at the top of your hips to drift forward, creating a tummy pooch in the front and tension in your lower back. The exercises in LBN will fix that by lengthening your hip flexors and activating muscles in your butt.

• **Flat bottoms.** Why do our bottoms sag? Because the average woman uses her quads more than her glutes. This program will get your tush firing again and literally wake your butt up.

• **Unstable cores.** All those crunches you've been doing since those long-ago PE classes haven't actually been flattening your mid-section. (What's more, they might actually be shortening your hip flexors.) Instead, LBN will focus on exercises that *stabilize* your core. Translation: **zero crunches!**

solid *to the* core

▶▶ Want to tap the belly-blasting power of Pilates on your do-anything day? Start with these five basic exercises from Michele S. Olson, PhD.

Ab Prep

1. Lie on your back on a mat, knees bent, feet hip-distance apart, and spine neutral—neither arched nor flat against the floor. Inhale.

2. Exhale, curling your upper body off the mat without pressing your lower back into the mat. Raise your arms slightly as you curl up.

3. Hold the position as you inhale.

4. Exhale and curl back down to the starting position. Do 5 to 8 repetitions.

Pilates Hundred with Knees Bent

1. Lie on your back, arms at your sides, knees bent and feet flat on the floor. Inhale.

2. As you exhale, lift your head and shoulders off the floor, bringing your arms along with them until they're about ¼ inch off the floor.

3. Contract your abs, squeeze your pelvic floor muscles, and vigorously pump your arms up and down, keeping them straight and rigid. Inhale for 5 counts and then exhale for 5 counts. Repeat 9 more times, for a total of 100 breaths.

Crisscross

1. Lie on your back, head lifted, hands behind your head, and knees bent toward your chest.

2. Inhaling, extend your right leg until it's straight and at a 45-degree angle to the floor. At the same time, twist your upper body toward the left, until your right elbow touches your left knee.

3. Hold the position as you exhale, then inhale and switch legs, bending the right one and straightening the left. That's 1 rep; do up to 10 reps.

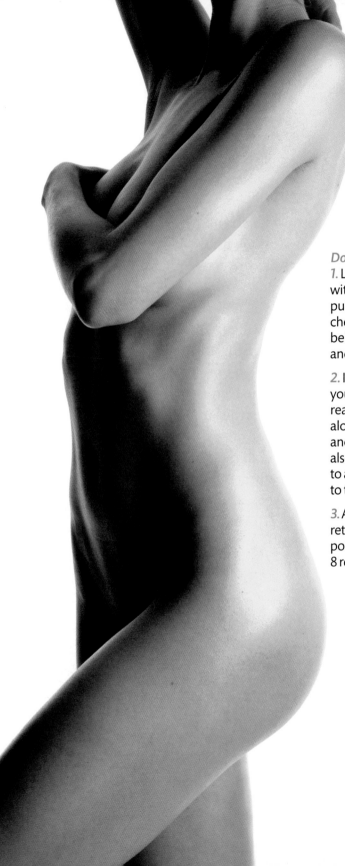

Double-Leg Stretch

1. Lie on your back with both knees pulled toward your chest, hands just below your knees, and your head lifted.

2. Inhale and stretch your body long, reaching your arms alongside your ears and overhead while also lifting your legs to a 45-degree angle to the floor.

3. As you exhale, return to the starting position. Do 5 to 8 reps.

Single-Leg Stretch

1. Lie on your back with your right knee bent toward your chest and your left leg bent at a 45-degree with your foot flat on the floor.

2. Place both hands just below your right knee and lift your head off the floor. Keep it lifted throughout the exercise.

3. Tighten your abs and exhale. As you do, kick your right leg out straight and bring your left knee in toward your chest. Hold it with both hands in the same position. Inhale.

4. Exhale and switch legs, and continue to alternate. Do 3 sets of 10 to 15 reps.

phase 2: WEEKS 4 TO 6

➧➧ You should have developed a sturdy base strength during Phase 1. You may have even begun to *see* some improvements in your body. If you didn't, that's okay. You're going to now! For this stint your repetitions will drop from 15 to 8, but you'll increase the amount of weight you're lifting. The exact amount depends on what you were using in Phase 1, but here's an approximation. Say you were using 10-pound dumbbells for your stationary lunges at the end of Phase 1. For Phase 2, use 15-pound dumbbells for the front-foot-elevated lunges. And, as I mentioned earlier in the chapter, continue to increase the amount of weight you're lifting each week by 10 percent, and remember to use the same basic crescendo I mentioned before—complete 1 set of each circuit in week 1, 2 sets in week 2, and 3 sets using your max weight in week 3. Notice, too, that instead of just going back and forth between two exercises like before, you will be doing two circuits that consist of three exercises each, and that the exercises will increase in difficulty. For example, Phase 1 called for incline pushups—you should now try to do them on the floor.

Be Patient with Yourself

Depending on your body, you may even require 4 weeks per phase. If you've skipped 2 or 3 days in Phase 1 and can't honestly say that you've "conquered" the exercises or workouts, stick with them a little bit longer until you do.

strength workout A

EXERCISE	SETS	REPS	TEMPO/TIME	REST
Dynamic Warmup	See page 106			
1A: T-Stabilization	1–3	8/side	moderate	60 sec
2A: Front-Foot-Elevated Lunge*	1–3	8/side	moderate	60 sec
2B: Bent-Over Reverse Fly*	1–3	8	moderate	60 sec
2C: Single-Leg Hip-Thigh Extension	1–3	8/side	moderate	60 sec
3A: Standing Alternating Overhead Press*	1–3	8	moderate	60 sec
3B: Reverse Wood Chop*	1–3	8/side	moderate	60 sec
3C: Romanian Deadlift with Dumbbells*	1–3	8	moderate	60 sec

strength workout B

EXERCISE	SETS	REPS	TEMPO/TIME	REST
Dynamic Warmup	See page 106			
1A: Prone Cobra	1–3	1	60-90 sec	60 sec
2A: SHELC	1–3	8	moderate	60 sec
2B: Pushup	1–3	8	moderate	60 sec
2C: Two-Point Dumbbell Row*	1–3	8/side	moderate	60 sec
3A: Split Squat*	1–3	8/side	moderate	60 sec
3B: Wide-Grip Pulldown*	1–3	8	moderate	60 sec
3C: Single-Leg, Single-Arm Romanian Deadlift*	1–3	8/side	moderate	60 sec

*Add weight as you progress in the program

1A
t-stabilization

start
- Get into a standard pushup position.

movement
- Transfer your weight to your left hand as you rotate your body and extend your right arm into the air so that your arms and torso form a T. Your right foot should rest atop your left. Hold that position for a moment or two and then return to the starting position to complete 1 rep. Do all your reps on one side, then switch to the other side.

Tip
Once this becomes easy, lift your top foot off the floor during each rep, so you make a rough X shape with arms and legs (as shown to the right). Holding hexagon-shaped dumbbells in your hands is another option for increasing the difficulty.

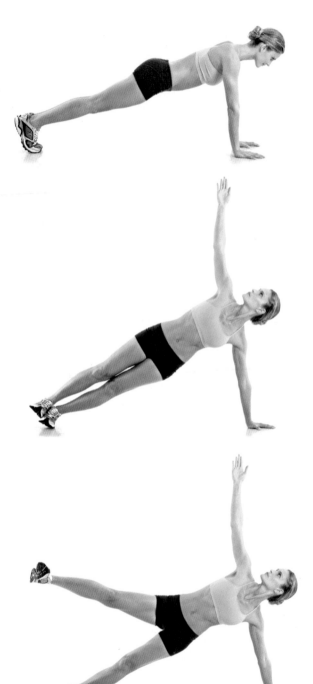

2A
front-foot-elevated lunge

start
- Stand tall with your feet shoulder-width apart and a box or small step 2 to 3 feet in front of you. Place your right foot on the box. (Having the front foot on a step increases the range of motion of the exercise.) Hold dumbbells to increase the difficulty.

movement
- Keeping your back straight, slowly lower yourself into a lunge by dropping your rear knee toward the floor. Keep your front knee tracking over your toes. You should feel this exercise in your quads.

- Go as low as you feel comfortable, and then drive yourself upward by pushing through your right foot's heel. Return to the starting position and repeat.

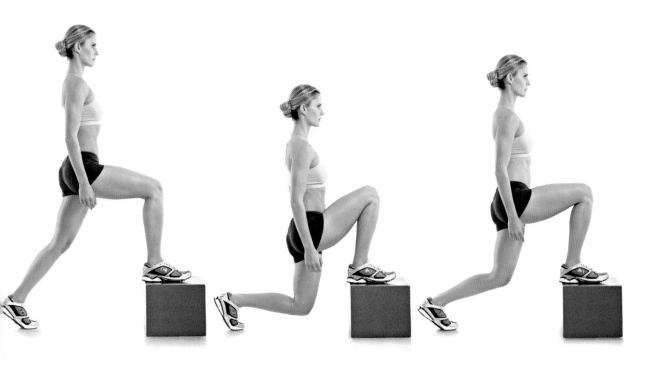

2B
bent-over reverse fly

start

- Stand with your feet a few inches apart and your arms at your sides, holding light dumbbells. Bend forward at your hips so that your torso is nearly parallel to the floor. Position your hands directly beneath your shoulders so that your arms are perpendicular to the floor. Straighten your back and tighten your abs.

movement

- Raise both arms out to your sides, squeezing your shoulder blades together. Lift your arms until they're parallel to the floor, and then return to the starting position. You should feel this exercise in your shoulders rather than your upper back.

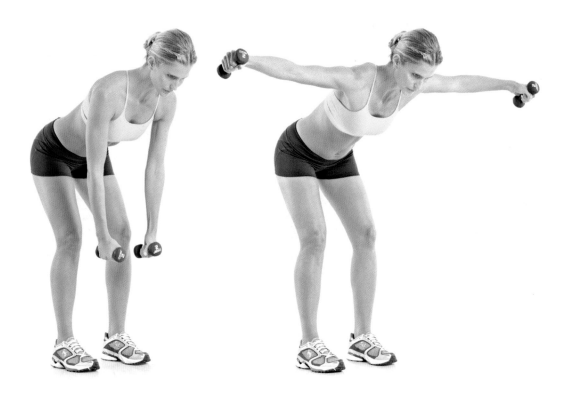

single-leg hip-thigh extension

start

- Lie on your back on the floor with your arms outstretched at 90 degrees from your body. Bend your left knee at about a 45-degree angle, so the sole of your foot is flat on the floor.

movement

- Drive your weight down through your left heel to raise your hips and torso from the floor. Keep your right leg straight and in line with your torso as it leaves the floor; your shoulders should remain on the floor.

- Continue to raise your body until your right leg is alongside your left thigh. Make sure your body is straight at this point and that both hips are even. Pause for a moment, and then slowly return to the starting position. Do all your reps on your left leg before switching to your right leg.

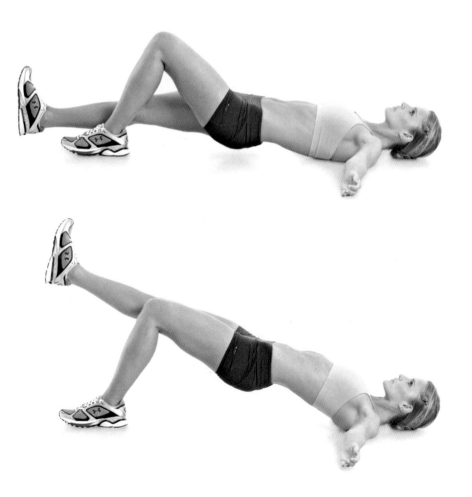

3A
standing alternating overhead press

start
- Stand tall with your feet shoulder-width apart. Hold a dumbbell in each hand with an overhand grip. Bring each dumbbell up so that they're alongside your shoulders, with your palms facing forward. Engage your abs.

movement
- Push your right hand straight up overhead until your arm is fully extended. Pause for a moment, and then lower it. Repeat with your left arm to complete 1 rep. Continue to alternate arms for the designated number of reps.

Tip
As you press the weight up, do not lean your body one way or the other. Instead, keep your torso perfectly still and straight.

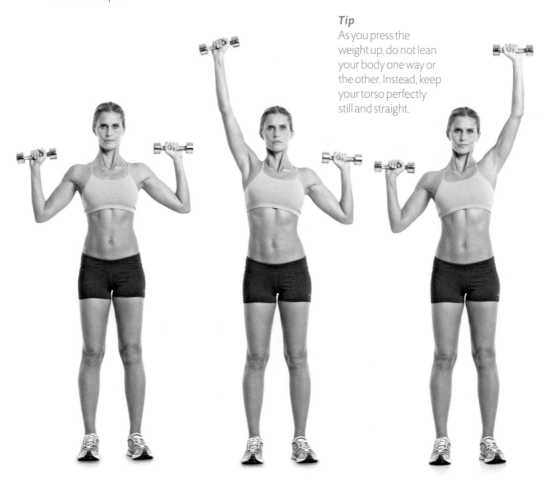

3B
reverse wood chop

start
- Stand with a pulley machine at your right side. Lower the pulley to the bottom. Hold on to the handle with both hands and straighten your arms.

movement
- This exercise is the opposite of the wood chop in Phase 1. Keeping your arms straight and keeping your eyes on your hands, pull the weight diagonally across your body from outside your knees to above your left shoulder. Return to the starting position under control. Do all your reps on one side before switching positions to repeat on the other side.

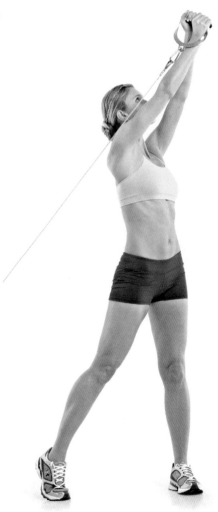

3C
romanian deadlift with dumbbells

start

- Stand holding dumbbells in front of your thighs with an overhand grip. Your feet should be shoulder-width apart with your feet flat on the ground. Bend your knees slightly.

movement

- Push your hips back a few inches, keeping your back straight as you do. Bend at the waist and begin lowering your torso toward the floor.

- Lower the dumbbells toward the floor as you descend, keeping the weights as close to your body as you can. You'll feel a stretch in your hamstrings. Go as low as you can, pause for a moment, and then slowly return to the starting position and repeat.

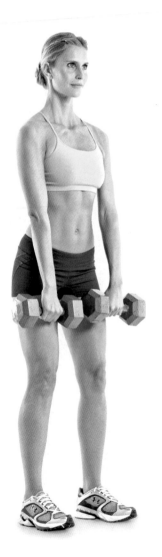

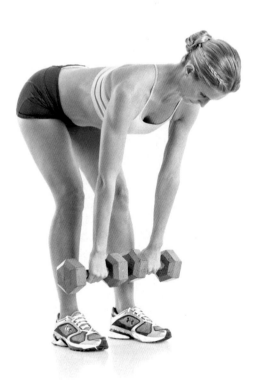

1A
prone cobra

start
- Lie facedown on a mat or carpeted floor and rest your arms at your sides, palms down.

movement
- Contract the muscles in your butt and lower back so that your upper torso and legs come off the floor. At the same time, rotate your arms externally so that your thumbs end up pointed toward the ceiling. Keep a neutral neck alignment. Hold this position. If you still cannot hold for the desired time, regress the exercise by doing multiple reps of a 5- to 10-second hold.

Tip
As you get stronger, advance to lying on a Swiss ball instead.

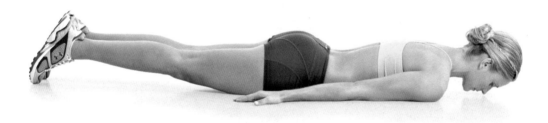

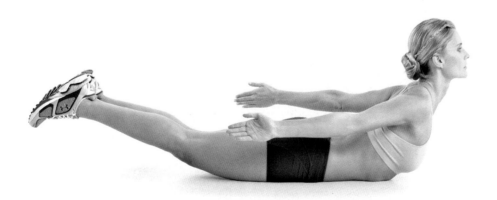

2A
s.h.e.l.c. (supinated hip extension with a leg curl)

start

- Lie on the floor with your calves on a Swiss ball and your legs straight. Place your arms out to your sides with your palms up.

movement

- Raise your hips so that your body forms a straight line from your feet through your hips to your shoulders.

- Now bend your knees and curl the ball underneath you. As you do, your hips should remain in line with your shoulders and knees.

- Keeping your hips elevated, slowly straighten your legs. Slowly lower your hips to the floor to complete 1 rep. Repeat.

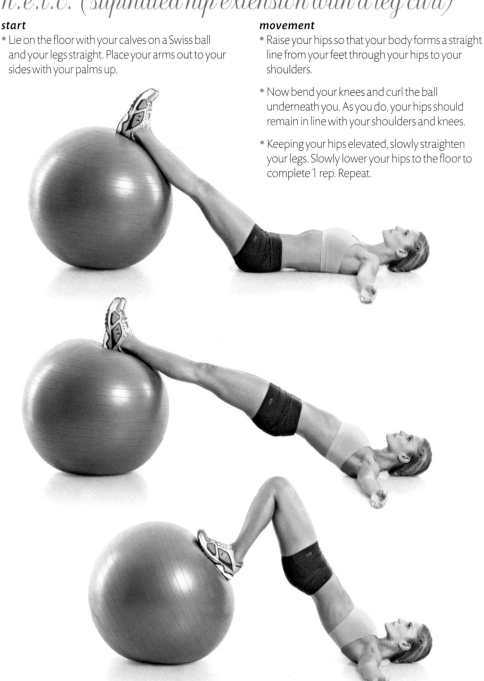

2B
pushup

start
- Get into a standard pushup position with your palms flat on the floor and your spine in a straight line, keeping your head, upper back, and tailbone in alignment. Don't let your hips sag or your back arch.

movement
- Keeping your abdominals tight, bend your elbows and lower your entire body in a straight line toward the floor. Lower yourself until your shoulders go just below your elbows. Return to the starting position, still keeping your body in a straight line.

Tip
Continue to rest your hands on an elevated surface if using the floor proves too difficult.

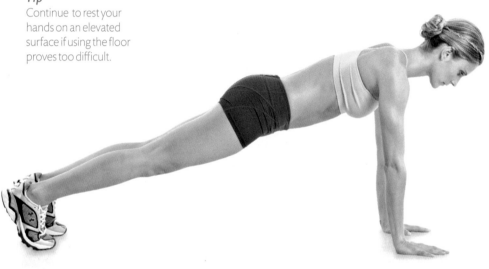

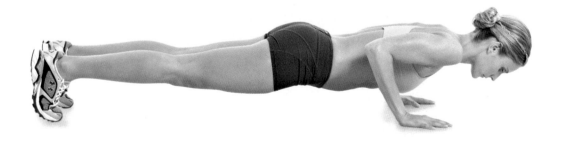

2C
two-point dumbbell row

start

• Stand with your feet together and your arms at your sides. Hold a dumbbell in your right hand. Bend forward at your hips, keeping your back flat and your spine in a straight line. Hold the dumbbell with a straight arm that's perpendicular to your body.

movement

• Bring the dumbbell to your body, bending your elbow and squeezing your shoulder blades together. Return to the starting position. Do all your reps with your right arm before switching to your left arm.

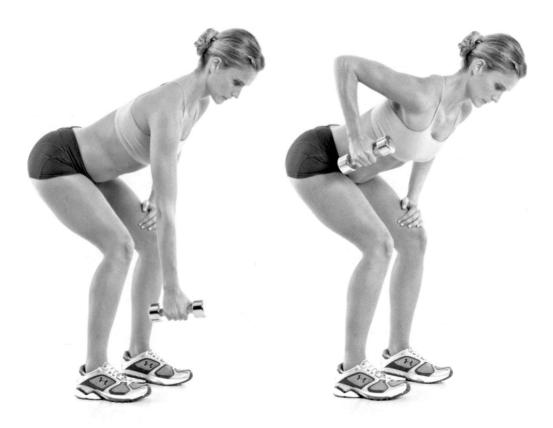

3A
split squat

start

- Stand 2 to 3 feet away from a bench, facing away from it. Raise your right foot behind you and place it on the bench. You will be in a modified lunge position with your torso upright. When you're ready, hold a dumbbell in each hand.

movement

- With the majority of your body weight on your left leg, bend your left knee until your thigh is below parallel to the floor. Your right knee should graze the floor, but keep your weight on your left leg. Pause for a moment in this position, and then return to the starting position. Complete the desired number of reps and then switch sides.

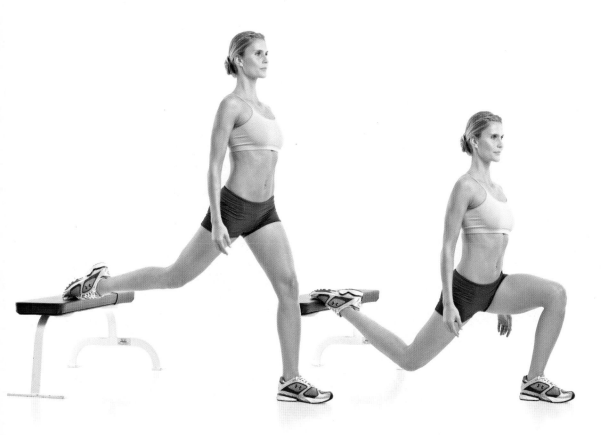

3B
wide-grip pulldown

start
- Sit at a pulldown machine. With your chest lifted and stomach tight, grab the bar or handles with your palms facing away from you and spaced several inches wider than your shoulders. Fully extend your arms.

movement
- Pull the bar down toward your chest. (It helps if you think about pulling your chest upward.) Bring your elbows to your sides and the bar to your chest, and then slowly return to the starting position.

Tip
As you progress, you can also kneel on a pad at a pulley machine, which is preferable, because it keeps your hips in extension.

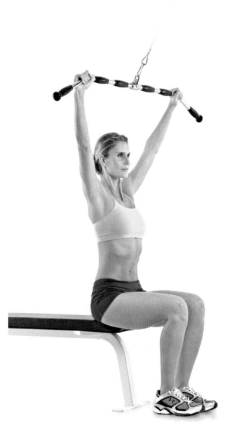

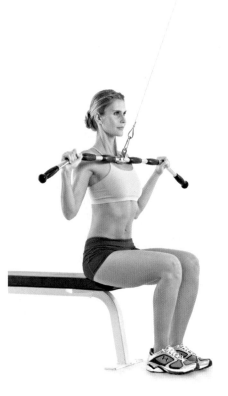

3C
single-leg, single-arm romanian deadlift

start

- Stand with a neutral spine; hold a dumbbell in your right hand using an overhand grip. Put all of your weight on your left leg. Raise your right foot slightly.

movement

- Push your hips back a few inches. Keeping your back straight, bend at the waist and lower the weight toward the floor.

- As you descend, raise your right leg behind your body. You'll feel the stretch in your left hamstring. Go as low as you can while maintaining a neutral spine—try to touch the dumbbell to the floor, if you're able.

- Pause at the bottom and then slowly return to the starting postion. Do all your reps and then repeat for the opposite side of your body. Add weight as you get stronger.

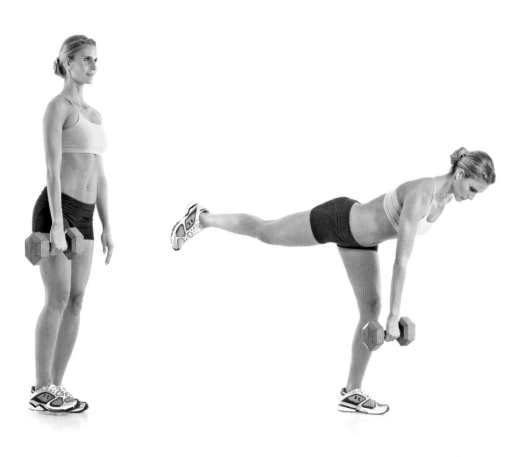

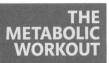
phase 2: WEEKS 4 TO 6

instructions: Do each exercise as many times as you can in 40 seconds. Rest for 20 seconds and then advance to the next exercise. Complete 6 rounds total, which should take you 24 minutes. Do not rest between rounds.

1A Sprint Run
1B Mountain Climber
1C Explosive Stepup
1D Static Squat In-and-Out Jump

1A

sprint run

start
- Stand in a room that's large enough for you to run back and forth, or stand beside an object you can run circles around, such as a barbell.

movement
- Sprint and change directions as fast as you can to get your heart rate pumping, or run back and forth or around the object for the allotted time.

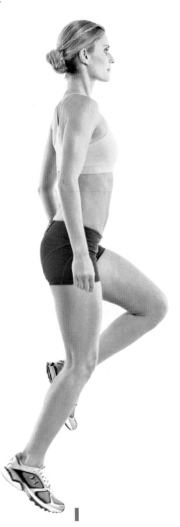

mountain climber

start
• Assume a standard pushup position.

movement
• Drive your right knee up toward your chest, then return the leg to the starting position as you bring your left knee toward your chest. Alternate legs as fast as possible.

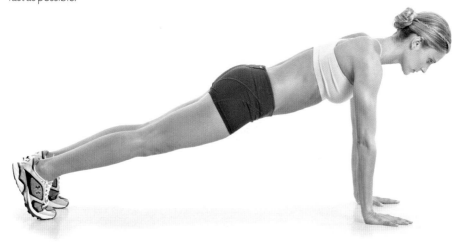

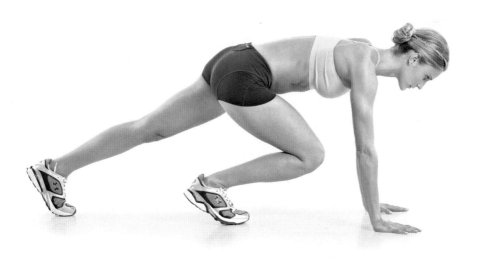

1C
explosive stepup

start
- Stand with a low step or box in front of you and your left foot on the step.

movement
- Put your weight on your left foot on the step. Explode off as you switch legs, and continue alternating legs for the allotted time.

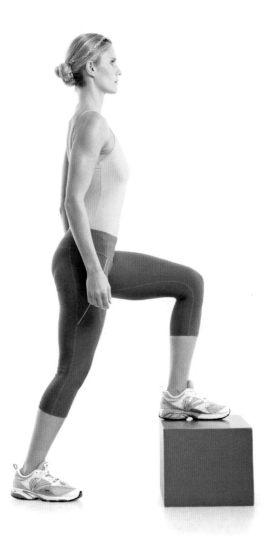
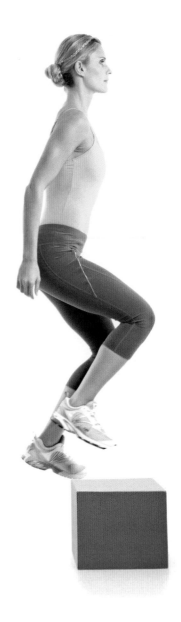

1D
static squat in-and-out jumps

start

- Lower into a squat postion with your legs slightly less than shoudler-width apart. Place your hands behind your head with your elbows back to enforce an upright posture.

movement

- Keeping your knees bent and staying low, jump and spread your legs so that you land in a wide squat. Then jump back to the starting position.

Once you've clocked 6 weeks of the fitness program, turn to whichever body-specific chapter you want to focus on for a new 3-week, results-guaranteed workout.

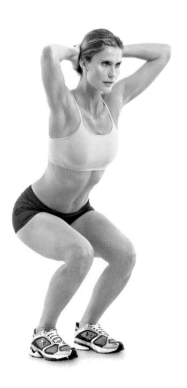

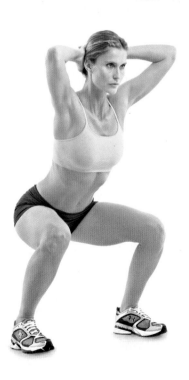

#1 Just show up

On low-energy days, head to the gym with the promise that you can leave after you finish your warmup. "Tell yourself you'll just do the Dynamic Warmup," says Rachel Cosgrove, author of *The Female Body Breakthrough* and creator of the Look Better Naked fitness program. "Once you get to the gym and get your blood pumping, chances are you'll finish your full workout. Ninety percent of the time, my clients do."

#2 Play the percentages

Have your body-fat level measured early in the program and then toward the end to gauge your fitness progress. "You'll actually have numbers that you can shoot for, and something that you can definitely measure, as opposed to, 'I just want my abs to look better,'" says Tim Kuebler, a certified trainer in Kansas City, Missouri. A body-fat percentage from the high teens to the mid-20s is considered healthy for most women (ranges vary by age), according to the American College of Sports Medicine. A trainer can estimate your percentage using calipers, and most gyms offer this service for a minimal charge; just have the same person do it each time, as measurement techniques can vary.

16 ways
to stick to your workout

(For those days when you'd rather eat nails than exercise, these expert tips will keep you motivated.)

#3 Book it

"You'll never find the time—you've got to make the time," says Chuck Wolf, manager of sport science and human performance at the USA Triathlon National Training Center in Clermont, Florida. While that seems obvious, lack of planning continues to be the biggest reason people fail to work out, Wolf says. He suggests keeping a calendar and your scheduling workouts at least a week in advance.

Have a contingency plan, too, in case the unexpected cancels your workout. "You're 40 percent more likely to work out if you have strategies to help you overcome the obstacles," says Rod Dishman, PhD, an exercise scientist at the University of Georgia.

#4 Make a date with a friend

Having a pal waiting for you at the gym will get you there. "If you've made a commitment to someone, you have a tendency to keep it," says Tristan Gale, an Olympic gold medalist. But that doesn't necessarily mean your best friend is also your best workout partner. Look for someone who's on the same fitness level and has similar goals.

#5

Target your heart

Heart disease is the number one killer of women, claiming 500,000 lives each year, according to the American Heart Association. Find out what your cholesterol levels are and what they should be. Then work toward meeting that target by exercising regularly. "You'll decrease your risk of heart disease while providing yourself with a very important, concrete goal," says John Thyfault, PhD, an assistant professor of internal medicine at the University of Missouri-Columbia.

#6

Be defensive

Need more inspiration than trimming your waistline? On your do-anything day, consider taking a self-defense class, which will increase your confidence as well as your heart rate. Learning practical defense skills—eye strikes, heel palms, knees to the groin—will also bolster your sense of control, says Dana Schwartz, a self-defense instructor. "You get to fight every class, and every class you see improvement in yourself," Schwartz says. "I think people are surprised by how powerful they are."

#7 Invest in a trainer

If you don't know what you're doing when you get to the gym, it pays to hire someone who does. Beyond helping you plan your workout, a personal trainer will observe and correct your form to make sure you produce results and avoid injuries. "They'll spot you through the movements, so you can really feel what muscles [are working]," says Brenda Powell, a certified trainer and general manager of the Institute of Human Performance in Boca Raton, Florida.

#8 Find a happy place

You hate fish, but that doesn't mean you stop eating. The same is true for exercise. "I can recommend running," says Ronald W. Deitrick, PhD, director of exercise science at the University of Scranton. "But if a person doesn't like running they're not going to do it. They don't care what the benefit is." The "perfect" exercise is the one you're happiest doing, so make sure you find yourself *wanting* to work out.

#9 Watch the rut

You found the perfect routine—great. Just don't let it become as familiar as *Friends* reruns. What bores your mind also bores your body. You need variety to guarantee results, which is why the Look Better Naked fitness routine varies day to day and completely changes every 3 weeks. If you did the same 3-sets-of-8 circuit week after week, you'd stop challenging your body around Week 4, and progress would plateau. "When you impose a stress on your body, your body adapts to it," says exercise physiologist Tom Holland.

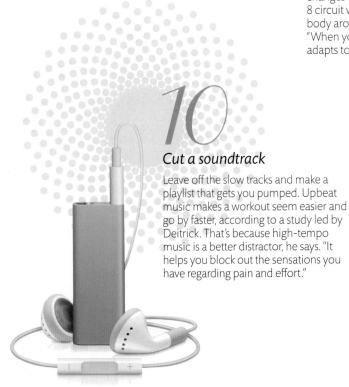

#10 Cut a soundtrack

Leave off the slow tracks and make a playlist that gets you pumped. Upbeat music makes a workout seem easier and go by faster, according to a study led by Deitrick. That's because high-tempo music is a better distractor, he says. "It helps you block out the sensations you have regarding pain and effort."

#11 Write it down

Record your fitness goals in a journal and track your workouts. Include the usual stats, such as specific exercises, duration, weight, sets, and reps. Write down your perceptions, too. "Think: 'Am I having fun, or does it feel like work?'" says Sara Ivanhoe, instructor of the *Yoga for Dummies* series. Note the exercises that make you feel good and produce results, and note the stressors that tend to derail workouts.

#12

Work with him

A Duke University study showed that sedentary men are 50 percent more likely to work out three times a week if their partners participate. It'll strengthen your bond, too. "Eighty percent of couples who divorce say they grew apart," says Pat Love, EdD, a relationship therapist and co-author of *Hot Monogamy*. "Sharing activities is a surefire way to stick together. Especially activities where you both end up feeling good and energized." Exercise releases neurohormones that make people feel happier, more motivated, and less anxious, Love says. "And anytime you have a pleasurable experience when you're with your partner, your brain associates him with pleasure."

#13

Take a chance

On your optional do-anything day, boost your adrenaline with a workout that challenges both your body and your fears—rock climbing, for example. Besides being great exercise, an adrenaline-spiked adventure will help you better manage stress in everyday life, according to a study from Texas A&M University. Adventure sports raise your levels of adrenaline and the stress hormone cortisol, and also provide you with an immediate way—exercise—to efficiently work that stress out. The fitter you are, the study found, the better you handle stress.

#14

Streak!

See how long you can go without missing a workout, and then try to beat your record. "Every time your streak ends, strive to set a longer mark in your new attempt," says trainer John Williams.

#15

Reward yourself

When you reach a goal—say the end of Week 3—be good to yourself. Celebrate by treating yourself to whatever you want—that massage or long, hot bath, for example. But don't let the moment pass; sometimes that short-term reward might be the only evidence of your long-term success, says Jacqueline Wagner, a certified trainer. "Some of the things we see in exercise in terms of maintaining balance, of maintaining bone mass, of maintaining function, we're not going to see for years down the road," Wagner says. A Swedish massage, on the other hand, can make you feel good right now.

#16

Show off

A boost to your appearance—be it a new haircut or fresh-out-of-the-box running shoes—can give you a lift in the gym. "Sometimes those little things can be very uplifting and motivating," Wagner says. "And when you feel better about yourself, you're going to function better."

the finishing touches

Grooming tips that will improve
your looks from head to toe

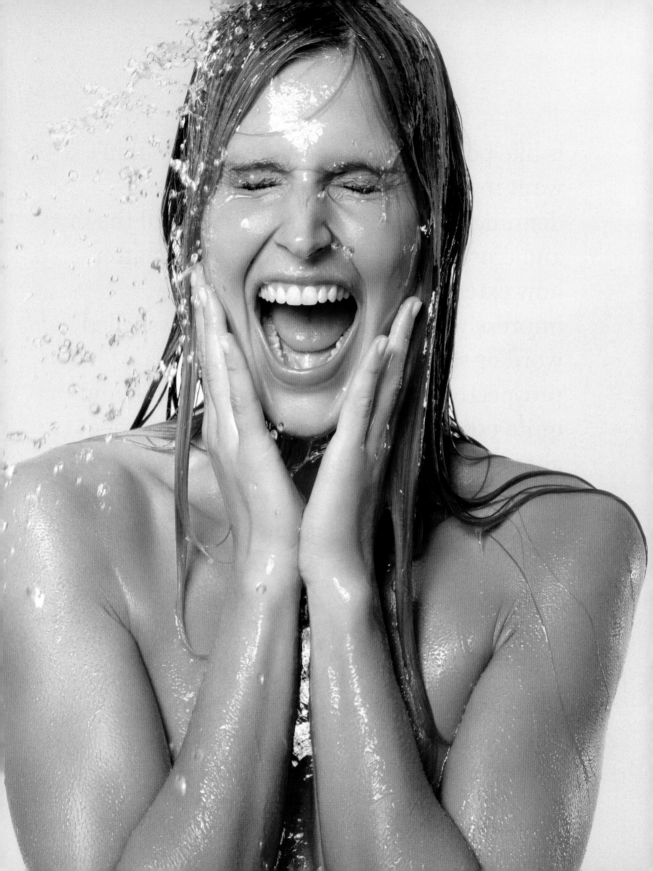

This part of the Look Better Naked program is like polishing your résumé. You wouldn't want to send out that all-important self-defining document without dotting all the i's and crossing all the t's—because no matter how extensive your education or how impressive your career history, a misspelled word or stupid typo will jump out at a prospective employer like a sore thumb and quite possibly make him or her think twice about considering you for the job.

I'm not suggesting that your partner will reject you because of sandpapery feet or fuzzy legs (or even a couple of errant nipple hairs). In fact, when face-to-face with a naked woman, most guys are going to see nothing but the "good parts"—the curve of her hips, the roundness of her breasts, the sparkle in her eyes, those big-picture attributes that he was attracted to in the first place.

All that said, when it comes to *feeling* sexy and gorgeous, little details matter big-time. If you put in the effort to sculpt beautiful shoulders but don't deal with the pimples sprinkled across them, you're bound to feel self-conscious, and the results of your hard work won't be half as stunning. If your slimmer, trimmer, stronger physique is punctuated by calloused feet and unkempt toenails, the effect will be all but ruined. If you let your body hair run a little on the wild side (no law against that, by the way) but feel prettier and more polished when your legs are sleek and your lady parts are tidy, it won't matter if you can bounce Ping-Pong balls off your belly, you'll have the nagging feeling that you've forgotten something—and that's going to be a confidence buster, I guarantee it. And as you know by now, viewing yourself as attractive, confident, and sexy is nine-tenths of the LBN law: How you feel is an enormous part of the image you project to others.

In this chapter, you'll find a wealth of tips, tricks, and techniques for addressing those aspects of your unclothed self that can make all the difference between looking *okay* naked and looking *great* naked. You won't need to avail yourself of them all, of course: If you aren't plagued by the aforementioned pimples, for example, you can obviously skip right over the sage advice for eradicating them. At the same time, though, if you've been searching for a way to finally smooth out those sandpaper-rough elbows, say, or pretty up your feet, you'll find it on the following pages.

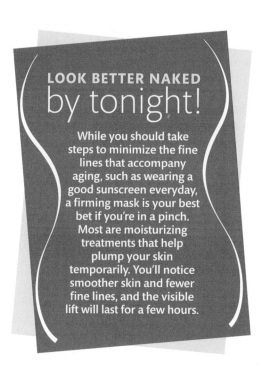

LOOK BETTER NAKED
by tonight!

While you should take steps to minimize the fine lines that accompany aging, such as wearing a good sunscreen everyday, a firming mask is your best bet if you're in a pinch. Most are moisturizing treatments that help plump your skin temporarily. You'll notice smoother skin and fewer fine lines, and the visible lift will last for a few hours.

5 shortcuts to a more fabulous face

Get a complexion to match your hot new body

Service your lips

The skin on your lips is highly susceptible to sun damage and dryness. Before you add lipstick, use a lip balm with an SPF of 15 or higher. Then, once a week, squeeze a pea-sized dollop of the balm into your hand and combine it with an equal amount of granulated sugar. Scrub the mix on your lips using a circular motion for a full minute. The sugar will remove dry skin and the ointment will nourish your lips and prevent cracking.

Let yourself glow

Dry, scaly skin reflects light chaotically, so that it appears dull. Slather on a rich moisturizer morning and night, and use a skin-brightening serum under your usual day cream to diminish dark spots and discoloration while illuminating your complexion. To improve uneven skin tone, use an over-the-counter lightening cream; those containing Sepiwhite are especially effective.

Win the wrinkle war

Skin loses suppleness when elastin and collegen, the connective proteins that support it and keep it taut, start to break down. You can't replace elastin, but products containing retinoids (which are derived from vitamin A) can boost collagen. In a 2007 study published in the *Archives of Dermatology*, researchers found that people who slathered on a retinol lotion for 6 months saw a 22 percent reduction in wrinkle severity. Ask your dermatologist about a prescription retinoid called tretinoin, the superhero of the bunch.

Be smooth

For skin that's both glowing and silky, first eradicate all traces of roughness by using a nondrying cleanser and moisturizer regularly. Look for a product that contains humectants, which pull in moisture from the air, and emollients, which smooth the spaces between cells. An at-home glycolic peel will also help, but if it's not potent enough, try an in-office chemical peel.

Clean your cabinets

Exposing products with a low H_2O content, such as lipstick and eye shadow, to water can hasten their decline. Kept dry, powders will stay safe for your peepers up to 3 years and lipsticks or gloss can last as long as 2 years. But gooey mascara has a surprisingly short lifespan: 4 months. Chuck it after that.

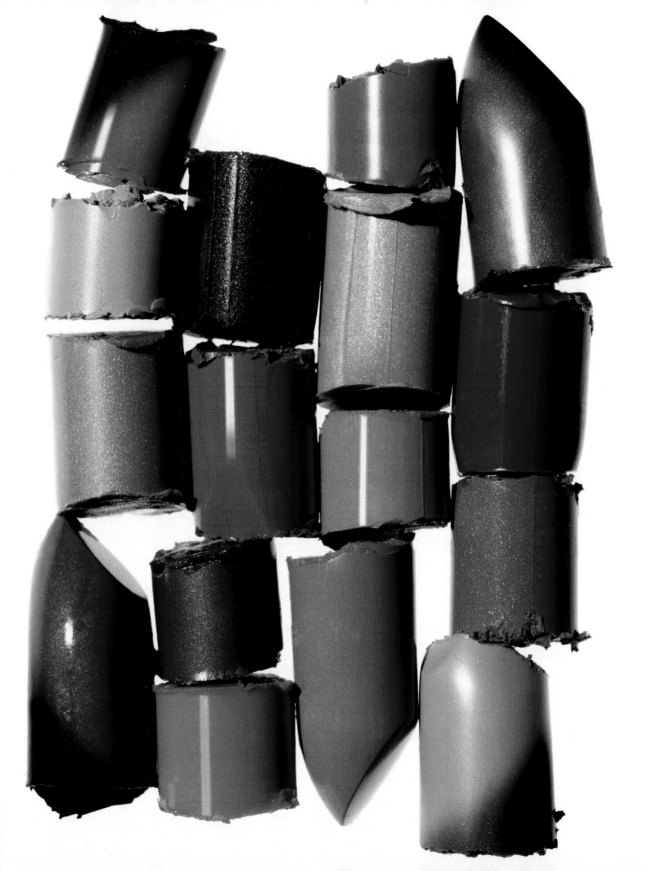

Beating Body Acne

Let's start with those pimples. Bumps that pop up below the neck are basically no different from the ones that pop up above the neck. Acne is acne, no matter where it takes up residence, but a basic understanding of the genesis of a zit will help you understand what's necessary to banish one successfully (and keep future bumps at bay), so here goes.

Typically, breakouts happen when the sebaceous (oil-producing) glands in the skin generate oil faster than the rate at which dead skin cells are sloughed off, explains Francesca Fusco, MD, an assistant clinical professor of dermatology at Mount Sinai School of Medicine in New York City, and a *Women's Health* advisor. This could be because of the havoc that adolescence wreaks on hormones, starting (or stopping) oral contraceptives, or simply a tendency to have oily skin. The overflow of oil gets trapped in pores, where it gloms onto the dead skin cells. The resulting mess not only stops up pores but often attracts bacteria, which in turn causes the surrounding skin to become inflamed and produce a blemish that can take on any number of forms, depending on how deeply embedded the gunk is. A clog near the surface of the skin usually shows up as a blackhead; if it's a bit deeper, it will manifest as a whitehead or pimple; the deepest blemishes tend to be super-icky lesions called cysts, which are the most likely members of the acne family to leave scars.

Acne can be one of the grosser obstacles to LBN success, but it's hardly insurmountable if you take the following steps:

• *Zap existing blemishes.* Pore-cleansing strips work wonders on blackheads, says Dr. Fusco. For the best results, rub the strip with your finger the entire time it's on your skin, until it's completely dry. Spot-treat pimples with an anti-acne product that contains either salicylic acid or benzoyl peroxide, like Patricia Wexler MD Dermatology Acnescription Acne Spot Treatment ($15, bbw.com); you can use a higher concentration—up to 5 percent—on the thicker skin of your back and butt. On your chest, use the same concentration that you would on your face—no higher than 2 percent. Salicylic acid often comes in spray form—such as Murad Clarifying Body Spray ($37, murad.com)—which makes it easy to apply to hard-to-reach areas.

• *Sweep away dead skin cells.* Exfoliating regularly guarantees there'll be less dermatologic debris around to mix it up with excess oil. If you like scrubs, you may find that a sugar-based one is gentler on your skin than a salt scrub. Tackle hard-to-reach spots (between shoulder blades, for example) with a soft-bristled, long-handled brush.

• *Address hormone-altering issues.* Birth control pills can sometimes help to counter hormonal upheavals that lead to extreme breakouts. You'll need to get your doctor's input on this one.

• *Tend your tresses.* If you're a sweaty-head type, yeast and bacteria from your scalp can piggyback on perspiration that travels down your back—a one-way ticket to a breakout. Corral your locks in a ponytail during workouts and wash your hair as soon as possible afterward. Using a medicated shampoo twice a week can help too, says David E. Bank, MD, director of the Center for Dermatology in Mount Kisco, New York.

• *Loosen up—your shirt, that is.* Sweat can get trapped under a tight-fitting top, and I know how much you've been in the gym lately. So if you can't shower pretty soon after exercise (or if you tend to get drippy in general when your heart rate rises), opt for workout wear that allows air to reach skin. Clothing can bring on bumps in another way, Fusco adds: For some people, the friction of cloth against skin produces a condition called acne mechanica. "It's especially common among women who wear thongs with jeans: The denim rubbing against the skin of the buttocks is the culprit," she explains. Deal with these blemishes just as you would "regular" acne, and consider putting a layer of silky, lacy, racy boy shorts between you and your denim instead.

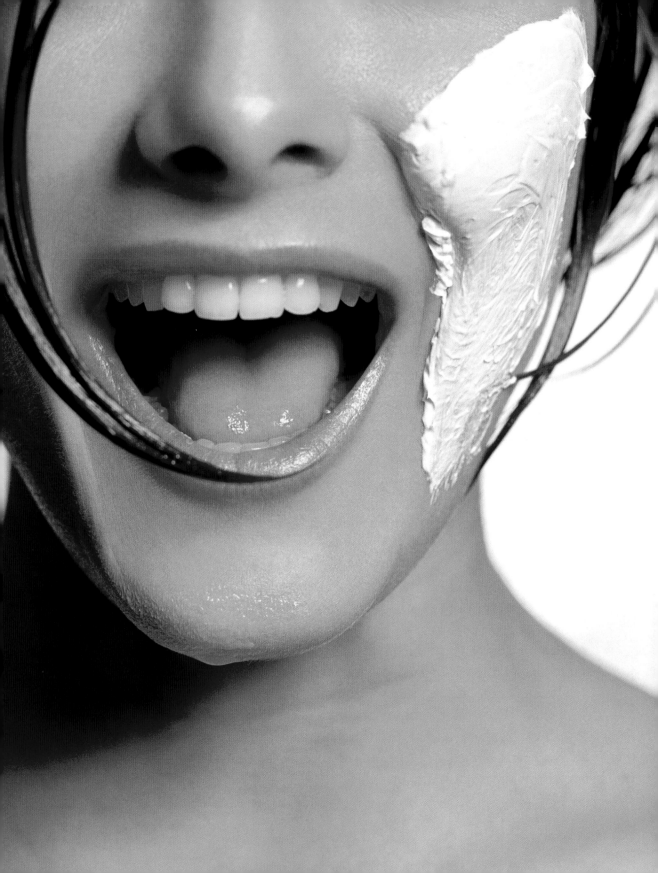

Smoothing Dry Patches and Rough Spots

Dry skin can look dull and flaky—hardly the most flattering foil for newly minted muscle. It can be particularly problematic in winter, when cold, dry air inside and out sucks the moisture from skin. Look for a body lotion or cream that contains glycerin, petrolatum, or dimethicone, Fusco advises. For an extra boost, choose a product that also has a hit of alpha hydroxy acid: It clears a path for the moisturizing ingredients by sloughing off dead layers of skin. Whatever product you use, follow these simple steps to get the most hydrating bang for your buck:

1. Shower or bathe first. Set the water temperature at comfortably warm—hot water can be drying—and try to limit your time under the spray or in the tub to 10 minutes, tops.

2. When you towel off, pat your skin—don't rub. You only want to soak up any rivulets of water running down your body, not every drop that's left behind. Your skin should be slightly damp.

3. Slather on your body lotion or cream of choice right away If you wait longer than 5 minutes, you'll miss your window of opportunity for trapping in the most moisture.

4. Pay special attention to knees and elbows. Elbows in particular spend a lot of time rubbing against surfaces (your desk, for instance), which causes dead skin cells to build up and create layers of rough skin. Lotions containing ammonium lactate or urea, such as Eucerin Plus Intensive Repair Body Lotion (which also contains alphy hydroxy acid to speed dead-skin-cell sloughing; $12, drugstore.com), are ideal, Fusco says. Rub it on every other night to soften skin and prime it to absorb moisturizer. On alternate nights, use an intense moisturizing ointment such as Aquaphor ($18, drugstore.com). And if your elbows are persistently dry and itchy, see your dermatologist; it could be psoriasis or eczema.

Another silky-skin saboteur is a condition called keratosis pilaris, a usually genetic condition that affects 42 percent of the population and is marked by areas of tiny bumps on the backs of arms, thighs, or buttocks. As with acne, the bumps are caused by a buildup of debris in the pores—in this case, keratin, an extremely strong protein that is a component of skin, hair, nails, and teeth (as well as the horns and hooves of animals). These bumps are especially tough to budge. You can't pop them, and forget pore strips: You might as well use Scotch tape to uncork a bottle of wine. Keratosis pilaris comes in two varieties: keratosis pilaris alba, with grayish-white bumps; and the inflammatory version, keratosis pilaris rubra, marked by red bumps, which some doctors think is related to eczema and allergies.

The number one treatment for keratosis pilaris is salicylic acid, says Fusco. Start with an over-the-counter product such as Neutrogena Body Clear Body Wash Salicylic Acid Acne Treatment ($7, drugstore.com), and use it every day, or at least three times a week. "It works, but you have to keep using it," she says. "If you don't, it'll come right back." You can also shoo away chicken skin (yes, it's sometimes called that) with an OTC cream or lotion containing ammonium lactate, such as AmLactin ($15, drugstores). It works best on damp skin, so smooth it on when you're fresh out of the shower. If you don't have any success with a regimen of salicylic acid and ammonium lactate, see your dermatologist. He or she may prescribe a retinoid or a topical antibiotic.

Dealing With Hair—Everywhere

How we women choose to groom the hair on our bodies can vary almost as much as how we style the locks on our heads. The only thing that's pretty true across the board is that many of us keep a standing date with our razors: According to a recent survey, 96 percent of women shave their legs, underarms, and bikini line at least once a week. And that number doesn't even reflect how much waxing, depilating, and lasering is going on in bathrooms, hair salons, and spas around the country.

Which brings us to the issue of which hair removal methods are best.

Ultimately, the answer is mostly a personal one: Whether you shave or wax, pluck or yank depends on what you can best tolerate, and chances are you've already figured that out. But some fuzz-busters can be more effective than others on certain areas of the body and for certain types of hair.

Shaving

The pros of shaving are obvious: It's fast, cheap, and effective. Plus, you can't beat it for convenience. You can keep everything you need right at hand, in the tub or shower stall. The cons: Even the closest shave doesn't last very long. Depending on how quickly your hair grows, you may have to shave every day—or close to it (especially in summer, when there's more at stake and hair tends to grow faster anyway). And shaved hair tends to look darker and more stubbly when it comes in than hair that's been removed at the roots (as in waxing).

56% of women say that they wear their hair "down there" neatly trimmed!

Because the razor shears each hair straight across, the part that emerges from the skin will be blunter and thicker than the tippy tops of brand-new, fresh-from-the-follicle fuzz. You also risk nicks and cuts, as well as ingrown hairs—but if you sharpen your technique, you can significantly reduce the chances of either.

Hone Your Technique
1. Start with the right razor.
Whether you use one with replaceable blades or a disposable, it's *vital* that the blade be sharp: "When you shave, the blade shears off a very thin layer of skin along with the hair; if the razor doesn't glide smoothly, it can take off too much skin," Fusco says—and you know what that means: red, irritated bumps and/or unsightly (and often painful!) nicks and cuts. After

you've used your razor (or blade) three or four times (or if you've dropped it a lot: Every time it hits the floor of the shower or tub, it can get a blade-dulling ding), replace it. Also, get a grip: Choose a razor with a nonslip handle, so that you can easily control it (especially around tricky areas, like over bumpy ankles and behind knees) and so it's less likely to slip out of your fingers.

2. Prepare for takeoff.

Research has found that moistened hairs require 30 percent less force to cut than dry ones do, so letting your stubble soak up some H_2O for at least 3 minutes before you go to work on it is key to a smooth shave. Shave with the warmest water you can stand—the higher temp will help to soften hair and open pores.

You also need some sort of emollient to further soften the hairs and to provide a slick surface for your razor to glide over. Let's start with what you shouldn't use: plain soap. No matter how lathery your bar is, it's still

What To Do About a Hairy Situation

If the landscape of your bare bod is marred by excessive, coarse, dark hair, you're among the estimated 5 to 10 percent of women between 18 and 45 who have hirsutism. Most likely this hair is on your chest, abdomen, or back (the face is often affected too). Because it's caused by an uptick in the body's levels of androgens (male sex hormones) or an oversensitivity of the hair follicles to normal levels of androgens, take this advice from the Endocrine Society and have a blood test to measure your hormone levels. The Pill, which suppresses androgen production, can help keep new hair from sprouting. To get rid of the existing ones, the most effective, least painful option is to have them lasered away.

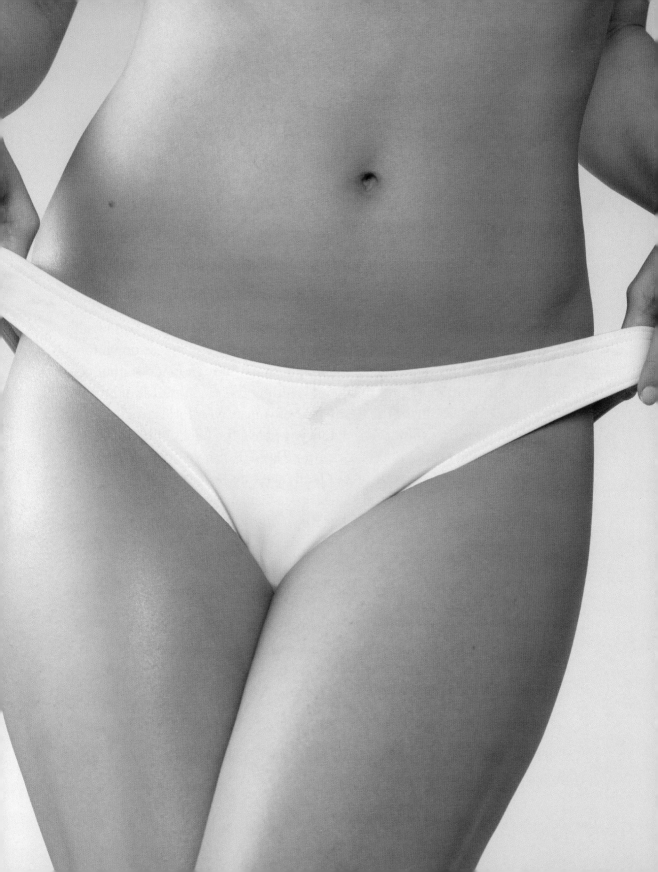

too drying for shaving and won't protect your skin. Opt instead for a shaving cream or lotion. If you're prone to razor burn, shave with an antibacterial cleanser, such as Dial Antioxidant Body Wash with Cranberry and Antioxidant Pearls ($5.50, cvs.com), recommends Ranella Hirsch, MD, a dermatologist in Cambridge, Massachusetts; it will help prevent infection that can result when the integrity of the skin is compromised. In a pinch, slather on a layer of hair conditioner: It'll prep the hairs and skin just like a designated preshave product will.

3. Know when to go with the grain—and when to go against it.

Shave your legs in the opposite direction of how the hair grows: from your ankles upward. Use smooth, continuous strokes and don't press down too hard—you should be using a clean enough, sharp enough blade so that you don't have to. With the hand that's not wielding the razor, pull skin taut in areas where it's least firm (the fleshy part of your calves, for example, and your thighs). Flexing your ankles while you shave the backs of them will achieve the same results in this nick-prone area. Rinse your razor after every few strokes. To rid your pits of hair, "start in the direction the hair grows, then rinse, relather, and shave against the direction of hair growth," says Myriam Zaoui, co-author of *The Art of Shaving*. Same goes for your bikini line.

4. Fine-tune your handiwork.

After you've given each body part a complete once-over, rinse off any residual shaving cream or lotion and check for hairs you might have missed. Any strays should stand out easily; a dab of shaving cream and a careful swipe with the razor will take care of them and leave you as sleek as a wet seal.

5. Trap moisture.

Once you're out of the shower, treat your legs to a moisturizing lotion with glycerin, petrolatum, or dimethicone.

Waxing

Waxing definitely has advantages over shaving: Because individual hairs are deracinated (pulled out at the roots), the result is ultrasmooth skin. This approach to hair removal has more longevity than shaving, too, because each hair has to make its way through the hair follicle before it's visible again. Most waxes last several weeks. One downer: Before you can rewax, you have to let the hair grow in somewhat, so that the wax has something to cling to.

The biggest potential strike against waxing: It kind of hurts—but not for long, and there are things you can do beforehand to soften the sting. And whether you do it yourself or go to a pro, it takes a bit longer than shaving. Here's what you need to know either way.

Before: Prepping for a pro job or a do-it-yourselfer

1. Do your homework. If you decide to wax yourself, make sure you get the right product for the body part you plan to defuzz. For example, the bikini area calls for a hot wax, which is stickier than cold wax and therefore more effective at yanking out coarse hair. Most products can be heated in the microwave. For convenience, buy a waxing kit, which will contain not just the wax but also spatulas for applying it, fabric strips for removing it, and sometimes after-care products. For hair on small spots like nipples and toes, try a cold wax, such as Sally Hansen Naturally Bare Waxing Strips for Faces and Little Spaces ($6, drugstores). To get the best pro wax, find a place that specializes in hair removal, one where the practitioner is licensed in your state to perform treatments; her license should be prominently displayed. And before you hit the table, check out

Sweet Relief!

Spas and salons that specialize in all-natural treatments often offer sugaring, in which a mixture of sugar, water, and lemon juice is heated to the consistency of honey and then slathered onto skin and used in conjunction with strips of cloth, just as in waxing. It's pretty easy to do by yourself with Shobha salon's Sugaring Kit ($30, myshobha.com).

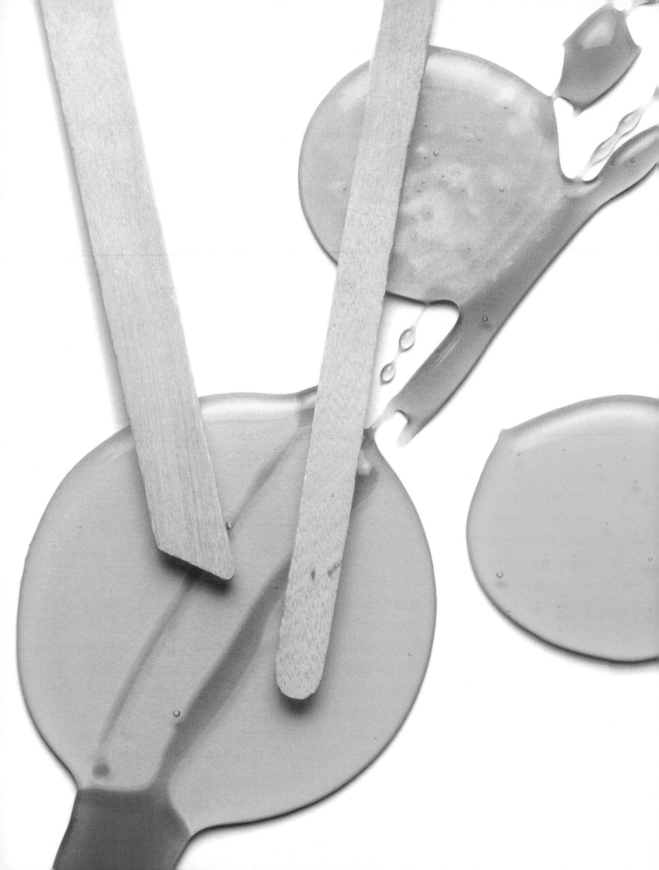

your surroundings. Make sure the instruments are clean and that the aesthetician uses a fresh spatula every time she submerges it in the wax: Double-dipping can contaminate wax with bacteria from one person's body that may then be passed along to another client's.

2. *Check your calendar.* If you're in the market for a bikini wax, schedule it for just *after* your period. Your skin will be more sensitive just before and during—plus it's more hygienic all around.

3. *Go to great lengths.* Wax will adhere best to hair that's about a quarter of an inch long. Let any that you're planning to wax off grow that long; likewise, trim hair that's much longer than that with nail scissors. This is especially important if you're going for a Brazilian wax, in which all the hair down below is removed.

4. *Get a jump on pain.* Fifteen minutes before waxing, smooth on a topical anesthetic like PFB Numb-It gel ($25, www.pfbvanish.com) or Relax and Wax No-Scream Cream ($20, relaxnwax.com). Two Advil about an hour before a wax can also dull the sting.

During: How to wax yourself

1. *Dry up.* Wax clings best to dry hair—meaning fewer do-overs and less irritation afterward. Lightly dust your skin with baby powder—as if you're prepping a countertop to roll out bread dough, suggest Cindy Barshop, owner of Completely Bare salons. The powder will absorb sweat and oil that even thorough washing and drying can't remove.

2. *Temper the temperature.* Of the wax, that is. After you heat it, test a bit of it on the inside of your wrist, says Barshop. It should be warm, not hot, and the consistency of taffy.

3. *Get directions.* Look carefully at how the hair you want to remove grows: That's the direction in which you should apply the wax. For example, if you're waxing your shin, you'll see that the hair grows downward, so apply the wax with downward strokes of the spatula.

4. Take it slow. Especially if you're a beginner, apply wax to an area of skin that's about 2 inches by 1 inch, and then firmly press on a fabric strip.

5. Don't be traumatic. Hold your skin taut with one hand while you pull off the wax strip in the *opposite* direction of how the hair grows—as if you're turning the page of a book, says Barshop. If you pull it straight up, you'll damage the hair follicles, which can lead to a rash. Note: If all this sounds awful but you like being neat and tidy, visit a pro.

After: Preserving your wax work

1. Clean it up. Even skilled shavers and waxers leave behind a spare hair or two. Prune strays with a trimmer designed just for that purpose, such as the Bliss/Philips Bikini Perfect Deluxe trimmer ($60, amazon. com): You can use it in the shower or on dry skin.

2. Soothe irritation. The skin on and around your lady parts is sensitive to irritation no matter how you keep it fuzz free, so this tip from Barshop applies whether you shave or wax down there: Soak a clean washcloth in milk and then put it in the freezer to use as a cold compress after shaving or waxing. "The milk is soothing and an anti-inflammatory," she says. For a few days following a wax, you can also apply an over-the-counter topical antibiotic cream and 1 percent hydrocortisone cream to ease irritation and ward off infection, says Bruce Robinson, MD, an associate clinical professor of dermatology at Mount Sinai Medical Center in New York City.

3. Prevent ingrown hairs. These are new ones that get blocked by dead skin as they try to break out of the follicle. Unearth them by exfoliating with either a gentle body scrub or a skin toner that contains salicylic or glycolic acid, says Hirsch. Try one that's formulated to battle breakouts, such as Clean & Clear Deep Cleaning Astringent ($4.50, cleanandclear.com).

4. Keep new sprouts at bay. Try a product with Capislow, a plant extract that's been shown to inhibit hair growth. In one study, it reduced the density of hair by as much as 50 percent after 28 days. Noxzema's Soothe and Smooth Refreshing Bikini Spray ($3, drugstores) has it; so does Completely Bare's Completely Smooth ($42, completelybare.com).

5. Cool it. Hold off on taking a hot bath for at least 2 hours, and stay out of the sauna or steam room (and, alas, avoid steamy sex) for at least 48, says Jennifer Pesch, brand director at Shobha Spas in New York City.

Let the Laser Do the Work

If futzing with razors or waxing is too time-consuming for you, there is a way to say sayonara to body hair permanently: with lasers, which use light to destroy individual hair follicles. The light is attracted to hair's melanin, the pigment-producing substance that's also responsible for the color of your skin and eyes. Lasers are most popular for facial and bikini-line hair, and they work on all hair hues (except for gray, which has no melanin), but the treatment is trickier on dark skin, since there may be less contrast between hair and skin.

A typical laser treatment will cover a 1- or 2-inch square of skin; it stings a little, but definitely not as much as waxing. The hair in the lasered area will fall out—forever—in about 2 weeks, says Cindy Barshop, whose Completely Bare spas specialize in laser hair removal. Expect to go back every 4 to 8 weeks in order to zap every hair. "Most people need more than six treatments," says Barshop. The cost: typically between $1,200 and $2,500 for the entire service.

Treating Your Feet

When it comes to grooming, feet often get the short shrift. Notice I didn't say toes: Plenty of women paint their piggies. But heels and other long-suffering areas often go neglected—and have the cracked skin, calluses, and other eyesores to show for it. More than half of women say they're embarrassed by their feet "always, frequently, or sometimes," found a 2008 American Academy of Podiatric Medical Association study. I highly recommend pampering your pups (and yourself) with salon pedicures whenever you can. Be healthy about it: Bring along your own clippers, orange sticks, and other instruments; some women even tote their own small tub to fit inside the pedicure basin. Preserve your pedi by massaging an überthick cream, such as Aquaphor, into your feet each night; in winter, when skin can be particularly dry and prone to cracking, slip a pair of cotton socks over your tootsies to boost the cream's moisturizing power.

Giving yourself a pedicure isn't all that hard to do:

1. Remove your old polish.

2. Fill a tub with warm water; add a foot soak, such as Earth Therapeutics' Tea Tree Oil Foot Soak ($8, earththerapeutics.com); or concoct your own: To the water add 1 teaspoon of tea tree oil (to banish stinky bacteria), a capful of witch hazel (to cleanse and tone), a $1/2$ cup of Epsom salts (to rejuvenate), and three drops of peppermint or rosemary oil (to heal and freshen).

3. Soak your feet for 5 to 10 minutes.

4. To slough off rough spots, use an exfoliant with medium-size grains, typically sugar or salt crystals, and moisturizing agents such as jojoba or almond oil. One good option: Sephora Super Foot Scrub ($22, sephora.com). Massage a quarter-size blob into each foot, starting at your heels and working your way out to your toes and calves. Rinse with warm water.

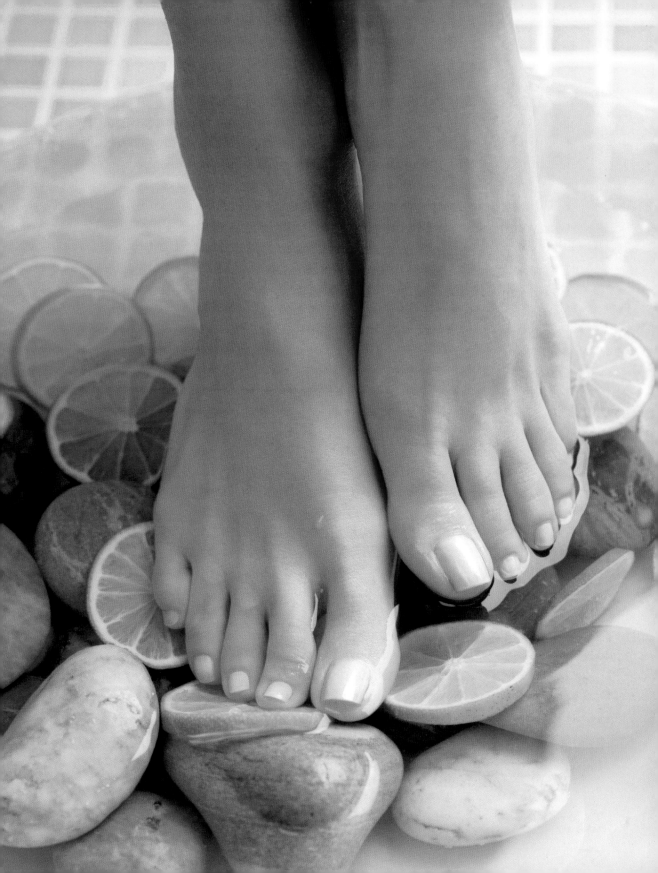

5. Wet a pumice stone or lava rock, and coat it with a little body wash. Using a back-and-forth motion, gently scrape your heels, bottoms of your feet, and toes. You only want to abrade the very top layer of skin.

6. With a strong steel clipper (try the LaCross toenail clip, $3; at drugstores), trim your nails straight across, then smooth the edges with a nail file.

7. Drench your soles with a product made especially for feet, such as Clarins Foot Beauty Treatment Cream ($25, clarinsusa.com); it has shea butter to lock in moisture, arnica to rejuvenate, and Laponite powder to keep feet dry. Massage a quarter-size dollop of cream all over your feet and lower legs.

8. With the knuckle of your index finger, press down gently into the arches of each foot. The mini-massage will relax your feet while boosting circulation, which reduces swelling.

9. Swipe nails with a polish remover to get rid of any cream residue.

10. Insert foam separators between your toes.

11. Apply a clear base coat containing protein, vitamin E, and/or calcium, such as Jessica Cosmetics Rejuvenation base coat for dry nails ($10, jessicacosmetics.com).

12. To apply color, start just above the cuticle of each nail and sweep the brush down the center of the nail toward the tip. Then sweep color on each side and across the edge of your nail. Do two coats; end with a clear topcoat.

13. When your nails are nearly dry, dab a few drops of cuticle oil on each one, to pump up the shine and protect against smudges. Boots Original Beauty Formula cuticle oil is a good one ($7; target.com).

R_x for Ugly-Feet Afflictions

CORNS AND CALLUSES

Look like: Raised layers of thick, dead skin on the tops of toes (corns) or on the bottoms or sides of feet (calluses).

Happens when: There's too much pressure or friction on the feet, often due to ill-fitting shoes or a deformity, such as a hammertoe.

How to deal with it: Once or twice a week, gently rub the area with a pumice stone until the skin begins to turn pink. Follow with a cream designed to soften calloused skin, such as Gordon Laboratories Gormel Creme with 20 percent urea ($12 for 2.5 ounces, amazon.com). If the layers are really thick, a podiatrist can shave them down during an in-office medical pedicure. Don't use OTC medicated pads containing salicylic acid, which can burn healthy skin and cause infection.

INGROWN TOENAIL

Looks like: A corner of the toenail digs into the skin, causing redness and inflammation. If left untreated, the nail can begin to grow extra tissue or drain yellowish fluid.

Happens when: Nails aren't trimmed properly or too-tight shoes squeeze toes so much that the nail grows abnormally.

How to deal with it: Soak the foot in plain, warm water four times a day and wash the affected area twice daily with soap and water. Keep the foot clean and dry at all other times. If you can, lift up the corner of the nail and place a small piece of rolled-up gauze between it and the skin. (It'll hurt, but it's important.) After every soaking, try to push the roll a little farther in. Call the doc if things don't improve within 3 days.

ONYCHOMYCOSIS, (AKA NAIL FUNGUS)

Looks like: Toenails turn thick and yellowish, or sprout powdery white patches.

Happens when: The fungus penetrates tiny cuts in the skin, or sneaks in under the nail during a too-aggressive pedicure.

How to deal with it: See your doctor. He may prescribe a medication such as Lamisil. To prevent future infections, keep your feet dry, never walk barefoot in public places, and leave your nails unpolished for a week every month. When getting a pedicure, make sure your salon sterilizes the instruments—or just do your nails at home.

the *look better naked* body menu

Tailor your workout to strengthen your weak points

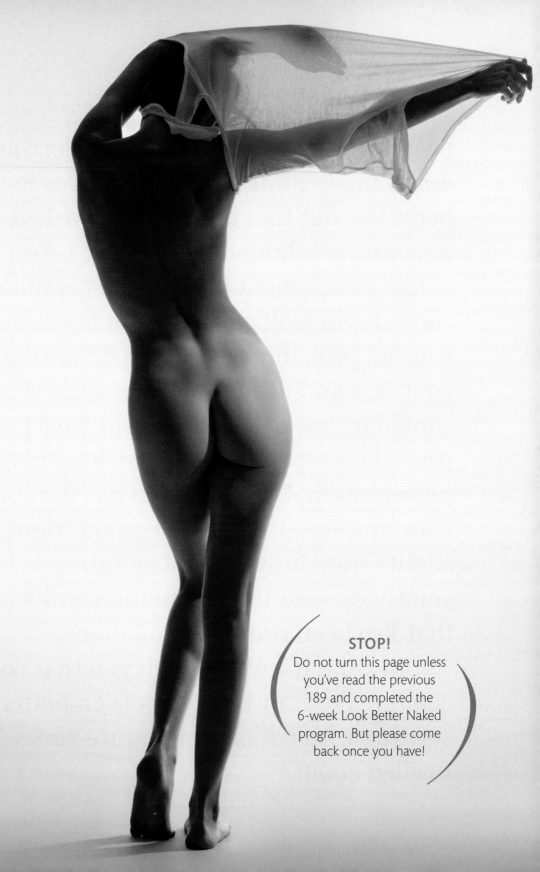

STOP!
Do not turn this page unless you've read the previous 189 and completed the 6-week Look Better Naked program. But please come back once you have!

If you're still reading this, I know that you've been working hard. In just 6 weeks you've no doubt made some thrilling changes to your body. Dig out that photograph I asked you to consider taking during Week 1. You look better naked, right? When you get out of the shower and look at yourself in the mirror, you can probably see muscle definition in your legs and arms. You've pushed your shoulders back too, which will have improved your posture and provided a perkier presentation. Your stomach has flattened, your butt has lifted—life is good, right? Right! Hopefully you're beginning to bare your body with the newfound confidence that I've been promising all along.

But what if I were to tell you that you could make your body look even better, starting with whichever feature you're least thrilled about?

That's right—you read it correctly! You've built a solid foundation over the past 6 weeks by torching fat, building muscle, and changing your mindset, and the following chapters are intended to capitalize on your recent achievements. The same weekly framework will still apply in Phase 3—you'll have 2 days of full-body strength training, 2 days of another metabolic circuit, and an optional do-anything day. Together these will guarantee that you keep your body in proper LBN balance.

Similarly, you'll still begin each strength-training session by working your core first. "Without strength there, you'll never get optimal results elsewhere," says Rachel Cosgrove. But in between your core exercises and your full-body exercises—which will be the same in each of the following chapters—you'll have an additional circuit that will target the feature of your body you feel needs a little improvement. Here's how it works: Pick the body part that you want to enhance—be it your belly, breasts, butt, legs, shoulders, or arms—and turn to the corresponding chapter. Within each you'll find four moves—essentially a customized circuit—that you'll simply insert between your core and full-body exercises for the next 3 weeks.

One thing to keep in mind is that different body parts will require different numbers of reps. Your lower body will respond better to lower repetitions, for example, while your postural muscles will respond better to higher repetitions, and so I want you to use the same number of reps for your customized circuit as you do for the full-body exercises. In other words, because portions of the workouts feature identical moves, some chapters will require that you do more reps than others. As in previous weeks, the exercises will again increase in difficulty as they progress—and pushing yourself will maximize the benefits. Continue to use challenging weights

53%
of women say that their men have asked them to get naked more often!

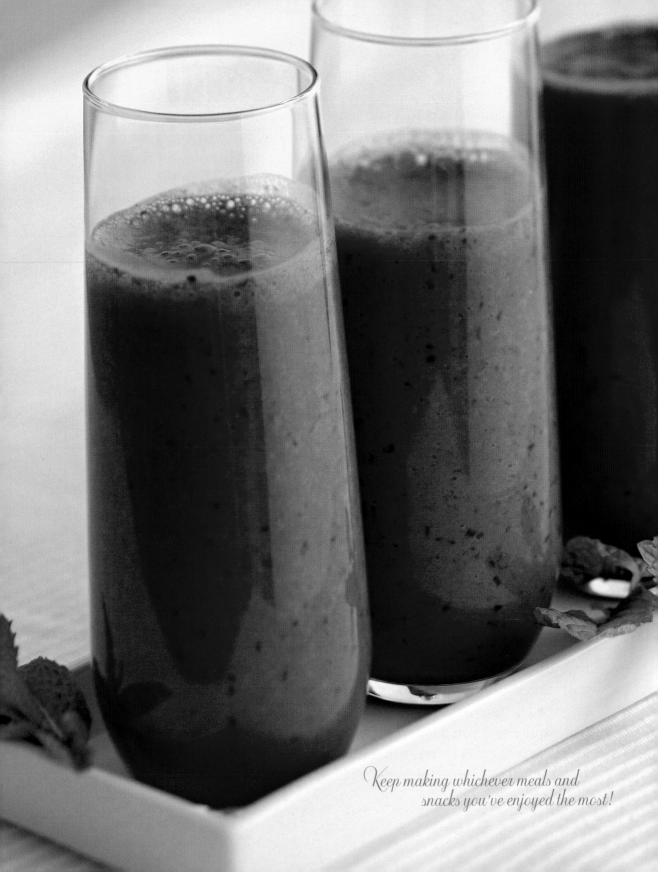

Keep making whichever meals and snacks you've enjoyed the most!

and to maintain good form even when you're tired.

An inevitable dilemma: You want to work on flattening your belly *and* boosting your bust. Well, if you have more than one body part to work on, you'll need to prioritize. "Focus on one goal for 3 weeks," says Cosgrove. "If you try to address more than one aspect of your body, you won't see the dramatic results you desire." The best part about this dedicated approach? Once you clock 3 weeks of focusing on one body part, you can advance to another aspect of your body . . . and another . . . and another!

As you ace your new Phase 3 workouts, I'll also have more risqué confidence-boosting ideas for you to consider doing in your birthday suit!

Lean for Life

Tart Shake
1 cup fat-free plain Greek yogurt
1 cup ice
½ cup frozen unsweetened cherries
1 Tbsp flaxseed
2 mint leaves

After 6 weeks you've hopefully discovered that, just as I promised, "dieting" doesn't have to mean deprivation. That's why maintaining your new weight shouldn't be all that hard—and why I won't tell you what to eat and when anymore. All you really need to do is keep on with a version of what you've been doing, says Keri Glassman. "You haven't had to count calories or anything else drastic," she says. "Going forward, you don't need to worry about that, either. If you're not feeling deprived, just keep doing what you're doing and follow a few simple rules."

1. If you want to indulge in something that's not on the plan, go ahead! Just try to limit splurges to once a week, and listen to your body so that you don't go overboard. Strive to truly taste your food—don't just stuff your face with a burger, choke it down, and move on to the french fries. Savor your sustenance, in other words.

2. If you're truly hungry—not just craving a treat or an extra serving at a meal—reach for something with nutritional oomph, like a piece of fruit or a small baked sweet potato. There's no reason to put junk in your body just because your tummy's rumbling.

3. Weigh yourself regularly: Once a week is often enough for most people, but if you're the kind of person who likes to keep tabs on your pounds more often than that, relax a bit. The point is to nip weight-creep in the bud.

3 more ways to feel Sexier

➡ Earlier in the book you discovered six ego-boosting activities to help you better appreciate your body. Now that you're already looking and feeling so much hotter, I'm going to let you improvise and come up with your own activities. It could be as simple as sunbathing nude or walking through your locker room without a towel, which 44 and 42 percent, respectively, of women I surveyed said they'd want to do as soon as they felt more comfortable with their bodies. Whatever it is, just commit to doing something that pushes your comfort zone at least once a week. And if you're feeling like you need a little inspiration, here are a few examples of women who overcame their anxieties and showed the world what they're made of—literally.

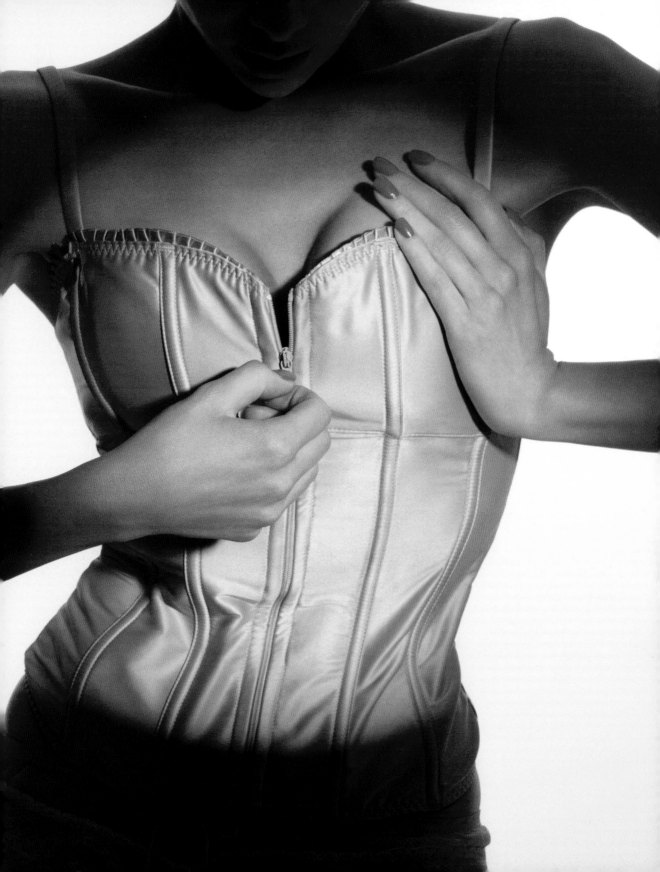

nude
awakening

➡ What would it be like to strip for art's sake? I liked what happened when *Women's Health* contributor Leigh Anderson found out.

"
Surprisingly, I found the dare intriguing: Model nude for an art class. While I've always been comfortable with my body, I seldom wear anything more revealing than a V-neck. So I figured it might be liberating to bare my flounder-white butt in public—especially in front of a crowd trained to appreciate classical Greek sculpture.

I called around and finally got the green light from illustrator Lynne Foster, who teaches a course on painting and drawing techniques at Pratt Institute in Brooklyn. Unfortunately, the night be-

fore, I made the mistake of watching a rerun of *Alias*. Jennifer Garner in lingerie, Jennifer Garner in swimsuits, Jennifer Garner in a onesie. Suddenly, I wasn't feeling quite so adventurous. What if the art students are so brainwashed by TV that they have no idea what a normal person looks like? I would really hate to be someone's rude awakening.

The next day, when I arrive at the loftlike building, I realize Lynne's class is all skinny young women wearing perfectly disheveled clothes. This makes me even more apprehensive. It's no secret that women can be harsher critics than men, who in my experience are usually just grateful to see any naked lady at all. I break into a nervous sweat as I start removing my clothes in a small storage room.

The two other models, performance artists Doug and Helen, have brought costumes to continue a theme they'd started the week before: *Cabaret*. They each don fishnet stockings, vinyl hot pants, black wigs, and white pancake makeup. I am not kidding.

Men are just grateful to see a naked lady.

I say a little prayer that the skinny girls will be kind and, clutching a long scarf, begin the long walk to the modeling stand. I settle in between and below Doug and Helen, my right calf tucked under my left thigh and my left toes brushing the floor. My hands are folded blandly in my lap. All in all, I imagine the composition looks like two deranged mimes and their naked pet. I can feel my face

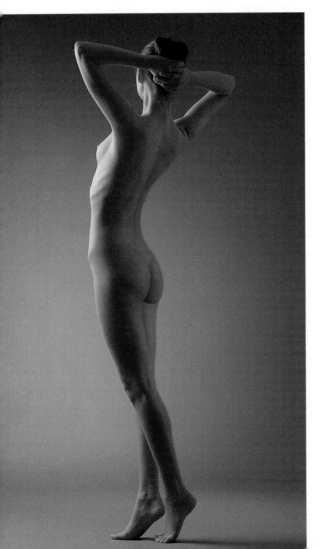

getting hot with embarrassment, but nobody's pointing and laughing; in fact, they have the same demeanor as undergrads everywhere—bored and a little sleepy—and as they start to scratch away at their pads, quiet settles over the room.

At this point, my thoughts turn to another typical feminine anxiety: Am I doing a good job? I resolve to hold still, to be the best naked pet I can be. For a while I'm torn between critically examining my thighs and hoping that I'm not twitching too

much. But as the 30 minutes we have to hold the pose creep by, nervousness gives way to discomfort—my foot falls asleep, my neck cramps, my nose starts to itch. I don't care about my cellulite anymore; I just want to stretch.

Finally, Lynne guides us into another position, with Doug and Helen seated back-to-back and me facing front and leaning against their shoulders. The skin contact is weird, but now I'm chilly enough to be grateful for the body heat. This 30 minutes passes more comfortably: Doug and Helen tell rambling stories, and Helen lends me her feather boa for flair. Just like that, I've been recruited into the cast of *Cabaret*, and the whole bizarre exercise feels a little more fun.

When it's over and I'm giddy with pride

for having pulled it off, I go to get my clothes. As it happens, I didn't leave them on a piece of unused machinery like I thought. No, they're submerged in a sink full of watered-down turpentine. As I stand there holding my soaked jeans, sweater, bra, underwear, and socks, a student walks in and stares—not at me, but at my solvent-soaked clothes. "Why on earth did you do that?" she asks. It's tough not to feel vulnerable when you're standing there stark naked, contemplating your latest boneheaded mistake. So I shrug sheepishly, pull on my cold, wet, stinky clothes, and hurry home.

As I race up the stairs to my apartment, the elated feeling returns—and it's not just from the turpentine fumes. With sketches of me in nothing but a feather boa now circulating the city, I feel just as fearless as Jennifer Garner. **,,**

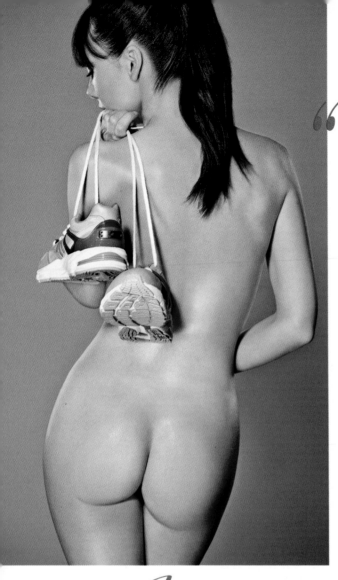

haulin' Ass

▶ Is there anything to learn from streaking? I asked _Women's Health_ contributor Blane Bachelor to investigate.

First things first: I am bashful about being in the buff. I leave my underwear on for massages. Lights-out sex is my favorite kind. Even wearing a bikini is pushing it for me.

Which is why, on this warm spring morning, I'm one sports bra and pair of running shorts away from a major panic attack. I'm about to do a 5-K. But it's not your run-of-the-mill race. Held at a nude resort about an hour north of Atlanta, this is the "clothing optional" Fig Leaf 5-K. (Apparently naturists, as they call themselves, are all about being comfortable.)

Why would someone so averse to baring her flesh sign up for this? I'm motivated by my boyfriend, Chris, an avid runner and the inspiration behind my completing six half-marathons, two

full marathons, and a handful of shorter races. Chris has run the Fig Leaf 3 years in a row and won't shut up about how much fun it is. Though I'm more interested in the bragging rights that come from going through with something so outrageous, at the heart of my decision is this: I love the adrenaline rush of a new challenge. But as the date approaches, I find the thought of my jiggling body increasingly mortifying.

On race morning we register and get our numbers—written in marker on our arms—and I say to Chris, "What the hell am I doing?" He laughs and casually peels off his T-shirt and shorts. Meanwhile, I wonder whether there's enough time to take a shot (or three) before the race. Despite a few lame attempts at giving myself a pep talk my nerves continue to rattle as we take our warmup lap. A few guys have already stripped down. I try not to gawk, but it isn't easy to look away.

I might be crazy, but I'm no quitter.

When I finally drag my feet to the starting line, I seriously consider keeping my clothes exactly where they are. A pack of 60-or-so runners—including about a dozen women, half of whom are fully clothed—is already lined up. I navigate the sea of sacks and cracks, careful not to make any skin-to-skin contact. When a volunteer shouts, "Thirty seconds!" I heave a deep sigh, yank off my garb, and toss it to the ground. It's a naked race, dammit! I might be crazy, but I'm no quitter.

The bullhorn blares and we tear down a steep incline. If you can picture how odd you look wearing nothing but shoes and socks, imagine how odd 60 people look while running in nothing but shoes and socks. There's more swinging and slapping than at a square dance. And forget about that "being comfortable" crap. My B-cup gals are jostling so much that at one point I clasp a firm hand over each and run that way for a few yards, feeling even more ridiculous.

"Want me to do that for you?" Chris asks. Hilarious. I glare at him and realize nothing about this is fun. Not the views of the runners in front of us. Not the way the naturists lined up along the route, mimosas in hand, cheer us on. If I weren't so uncomfortable, I'd be laughing about the absurdity of it all.

The experience gives a new meaning to the phrase "haul ass."

The 3.1-mile route is three hilly laps through the resort, and about halfway through it Chris and I have moved up to the front third of the pack. In just 20 minutes, I've seen more penises than I have in my entire 32 years. Every time we pass a runner wearing clothes, I have to fight off the urge to scream, "Cheater!" Focusing on others makes it easier to avoid thinking about how I actually paid money to do this.

As we wind around the final downhill stretch, I quickly grab my bra and shorts off the ground. As soon as we cross the finish line—at a respectable 25 minutes and 16 seconds—I put them back on. The award ceremony is held at the resort's pool, and after I accept (fully clothed) my second-

place trophy, Chris heads off in search of beers. Half an hour later, sufficiently buzzed, I take a quick look around at the expanse of bare bodies bronzing in the sun, and something inside me shifts. These people have already seen everything I've got, and at least now it's not bouncing around mercilessly. So I figure, what the hell? I strip off my running clothes and slide into the pool, loving how good the cold water feels against my skin—and how surprisingly comfortable I feel in it. Despite all those negative thoughts I had about it throughout the race, my body came through for me!

On the way home, I smile at my trophy. This one I've really earned, along with a newfound appreciation for my sports bra. **"**

center stage

➡ What can you learn from a professional seductress? I asked burlesque performer Ava Garter to reveal her secrets.

" **When I pull back my hair in the morning** and get my two kids ready for school, you'd never guess that I let my hair down at night and can make your jaw drop just by taking my gloves off. That's the beauty of being a burlesque dancer: There's more to me than meets the eye. When most women hear my profession they say, "You've had two kids! How do you have the confidence to do that?" Diet and exercise have something to do with it, for sure, but I simply love what I'm doing.

Burlesque is back in a big way, and I've noticed most of the audiences are equally divided between men and women. I think that's because burlesque is ultimately the art of the tease, and everybody finds something supremely captivating and empowering about that. My costumes are like a gift with an elaborately detailed wrapping that conceals the present beneath. A full 7 minutes will pass before I'm down to my bra and underwear, but the wait is worth the ... you know.

I also run a school of seduction in Southern California called The Black Glove. While technically I'm teaching burlesque, I'm really teaching confidence. And, as I tell my students, we need to do a better job of celebrating the special assets of our bodies. We pull our hair back, wear suits, and work in offices ... but then we may get down on ourselves when our boobs aren't what we'd like them to be or we weigh a few extra pounds. Yet we forget that men don't have the curves we do—and that they're in absolute awe of them. So learn to use them to your advantage.

Another thing: By birthright, every woman should own a garter belt and stockings. Our mothers and grandmothers cast them aside, told us they were pains, and we never bothered to pick them back up. Well, they're not pains. You just need to learn how to put them on—and take them off. Otherwise they're actually designed to make us feel comfortable and feminine. To me, wearing these elements is part of being a woman.

By birthright, every woman should own a garter belt and stockings.

Every woman should upgrade her walk, too. (I'm talking about the walk you use everyday—not just the walk you use to get a gentleman's attention either, although I like practicing that one too.) Watch women in the grocery store or mall. They slump their shoulders, curve their backs, and then scurry around ... terribly unappealing stuff. Why not have a really, really sexy way of walking instead? Just try to elongate your body from your heels all the way up through the top of your head. You'll seem happier and healthier, and you'll make yourself look like you've lost 5 pounds—no joke.

The other thing I do every single day is wear makeup. Even if I'm just dropping my kids off at school, I try to put my best face forward. You can handle almost anything when you feel good about yourself, and it starts with feeling attractive.

There's a lot more that goes into being a burlesque dancer, and you should check out my website, avagarter.com, or ask around to find some classes and shows near you if you're interested in learning more. Don't be intimidated to give it a go: The role of a burlesque performer is really just to celebrate her figure regardless of its shape or size. In my classes I emphasize

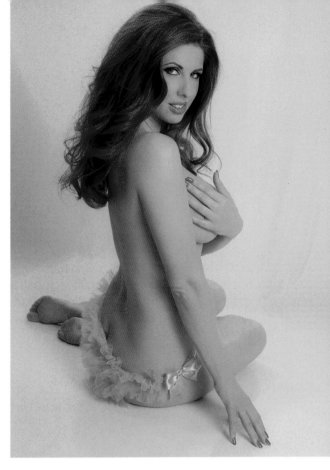

this by telling my students that nothing is sexier or more alluring than a confident smile. Eye contact is almost as important because it establishes that you believe in what you're doing and that you enjoy doing it. And the greatest thing about both of these is that you have complete control over them. Keep that in mind when you have a lucky someone on the receiving end of your first performance. I can guarantee that he's going to appreciate what he sees ... and feels. **"**
—As told to Joel Weber

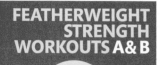
phase 3: WEEKS 7 TO 9

instructions: Use the following framework for the next 3 weeks, but remember to add the circuit included in one of the following chapters. You'll find the specific number of reps you'll need to do for the entire workout there, too.

workout A

EXERCISES	SETS	REPS	TEMPO/TIME	REST
Dynamic Warmup	*See page 106*			
Circuit 1:				
1A: Plank on Swiss Ball	1-2	1	60–90 sec	60 sec
1B: Core Stability Twist*	1-2	10–12/side	moderate	60 sec
Circuit 2:				
Customized Workout				
Circuit 3:				
3A: Hip Extension	1-3	–	moderate	–
3B: One-Point Dumbbell Row*	1-3	–	moderate	–
3C: Front Squat*	1-3	–	moderate	–
3D: Single-Arm Dumbbell Chest Press on a Swiss Ball*	1-3	–	moderate	–

*Add weight as you progress in the program

Wait, Where's the Second Station?

Don't forget to turn ahead to whichever chapter targets the body part you want to work on! That's where you'll find the details for the second station of the Phase 3 featherweight strength-training program. Insert those four moves here and complete them before advancing to the third and final station.

workout B

EXERCISES	SETS	REPS	TEMPO/TIME	REST
Dynamic Warmup	*See page 106*			
Circuit 1:				
1A: Prone Jackknife	1-2	10–15	moderate	60 sec
1B: Prone Cobra on a Swiss Ball	1-2	1	60–90 sec	60 sec
Circuit 2:				
Customized Workout				
Circuit 3:				
3A: Split Squat with Opposite Arm Overhead Press*	1-3	–	moderate	–
3B: Wide-Grip Pulldown*	1-3	–	moderate	–
3C: Single-Leg, Single-Arm Romanian Deadlift*	1-3	–	moderate	–
3D: Inverted Row	1-3	–	moderate	–

*Add weight as you progress in the program

1A
plank on swiss ball

postion

- Rest your elbows on a Swiss ball. Firmly plant your feet on the floor so that your body is at about a 45-degree angle. Draw your abs tight and keep your body in a stable straight line. This is a static hold without any movement—continue to keep your body in a straight line.

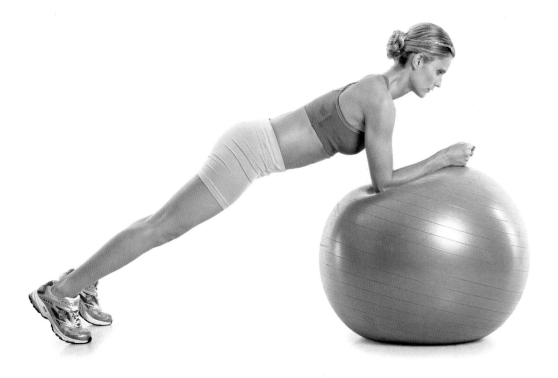

1B
core stability twist

start

- Sit on the floor with your legs spread apart, knees bent to form a 90-degree angle. Hold a small weight in your hands and extend it directly in front of you. Keep your arms straight and lean back slightly.

movement

- Keeping your torso and abs as still and as tight as possible, rotate the weight from side to side. When you return to center, that's 1 rep.

Tip

To increase the difficulty, lift your feet off the floor or increase the range of motion, the speed, or the size of the weight.

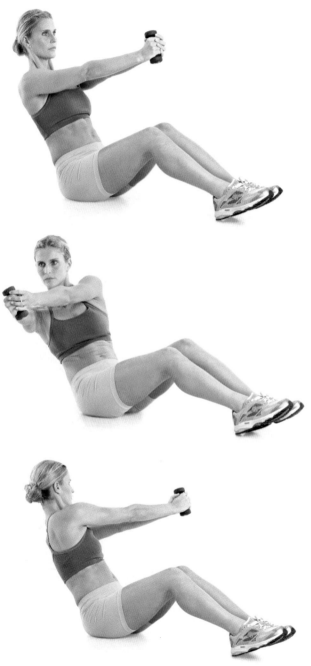

.3A
hip extension

start

- Lie on your back. Bend your knees so that your feet are flat on the floor. Place your arms at your sides, externally rotated.

movement

- Tighten your core. Now squeeze your glutes to lift your hips off the floor and toward the ceiling. Raise them until your body forms a straight line from your shoulders to your knees. Lower to the starting position and repeat.

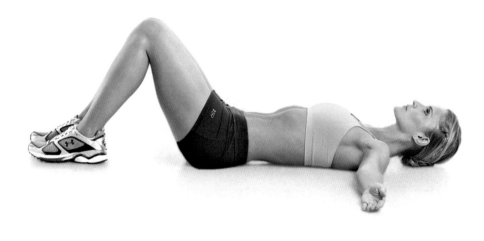

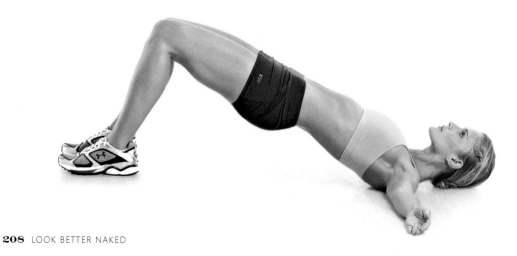

3B

one-point dumbbell row

start

- Balance on your left leg while holding a dumbbell in your opposite hand. Bend over at the hip. Raise your elevated leg behind you—use the floor for balance as needed—and keep your back straight and flat.

movement

- Row the dumbbell up to your side, squeezing your shoulder blades back and together. Return to the starting position while still balancing on your supporting leg and repeat. Do the designated number of repetitions and then switch sides.

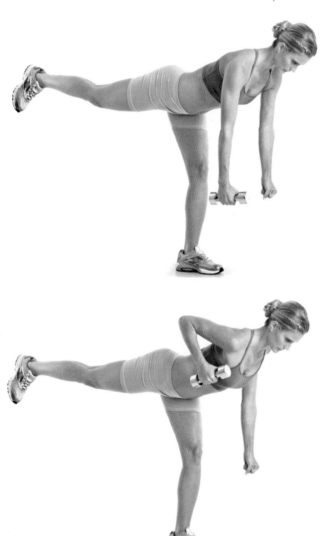

3C
front squat

start

- Using an overhand grip, place a weighted barbell across the front of your shoulders. Position your hands as close to your shoulders as comfortable and point your elbows directly forward. The bar should gently press against your throat and your upper arms should be parallel to the floor. Spread your feet shoulder-width apart. They should either be straight or slightly externally rotated.

movement

- Squat as deeply as you can until the tops of your thighs are at least parallel to the floor. Your weight should be on your heels, not your toes. Keep your knees an equal distance apart during the lift and don't let them drift forward of your toes. The concentric phase should mirror the eccentric phase.

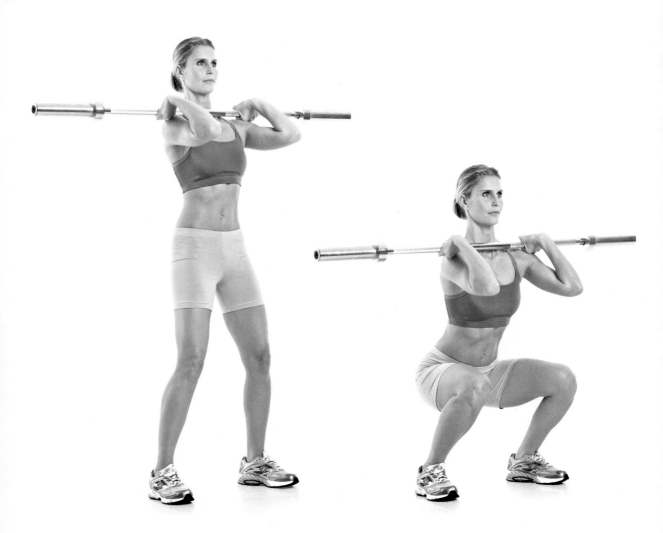

3D,
single-arm dumbbell chest press on a swiss ball

start
- Lie on a Swiss ball with your hips unsupported, which will force you to squeeze your butt and legs. Hold a dumbbell in your right hand about 6 inches from your right breast.

movement
- Push the dumbbell straight up, keeping your core flexed as you do so. Complete all your reps on your right side, and then switch to your left.

Tip
You can also do this on a Bosu ball or at the edge of a bench with your hips off the edge and just your upper back supported.

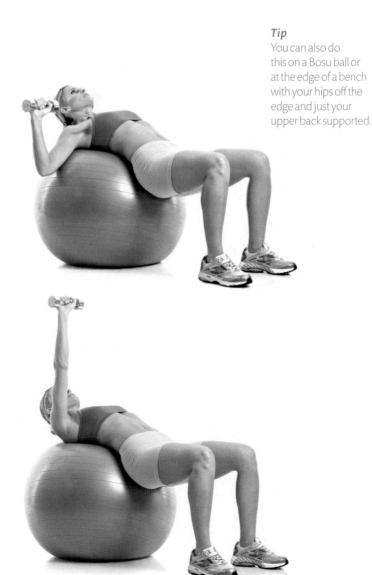

phase 3: WEEKS 7 TO 9

1A
prone jacknife

start
- Get into a pushup position with your arms fully extended and your feet on a Swiss ball.

movement
- Maintaining a neutral spine and stable torso, tuck the ball in underneath you. Pause, and then straighten your legs again. Your back and torso should remain still the entire time; only your legs should move.

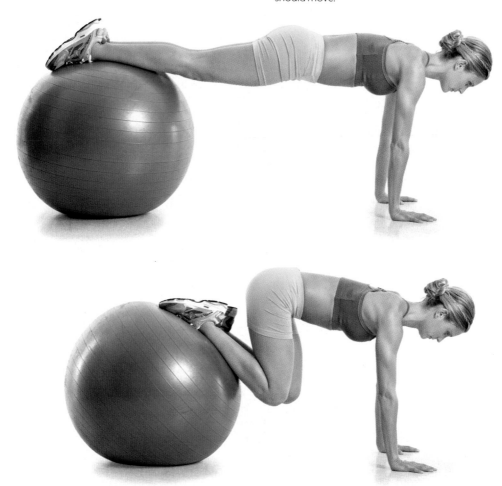

1B
prone cobra on a swiss ball

start

- Lie face down on a Swiss ball and rest your arms at your sides, palms down.

movement

- Contract the muscles in your glutes and lower back so that your upper torso comes off the ball. At the same time, rotate your arms externally so that your thumbs end up pointed toward the ceiling. Keep a neutral neck alignment.

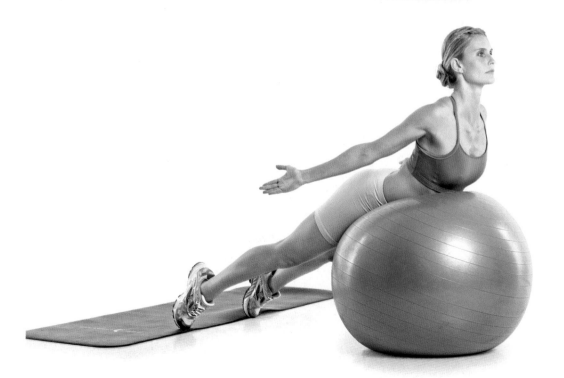

3A
split squat with opposite-arm overhead press

start

- Start with a bench behind you and a dumbbell in your left hand. Place your right foot on the bench and your left foot about 2 to 3 feet in front of the bench. You will be in a modified lunge position with your torso upright. Bring the dumbbell up to your shoulder.

movement

- With the bulk of your body weight on your front leg, bend your front knee until your thigh is below parallel and the knee of your trailing leg is grazing the floor. Keep your weight on the front leg.

- As you are lowering yourself, press the dumbbell overhead. Pause at the bottom of the lunge with your left arm fully extended and then return to a fully upright stance as you lower the dumbbell back to your shoulder. That's one rep. Repeat for the designated number of reps and then switch sides.

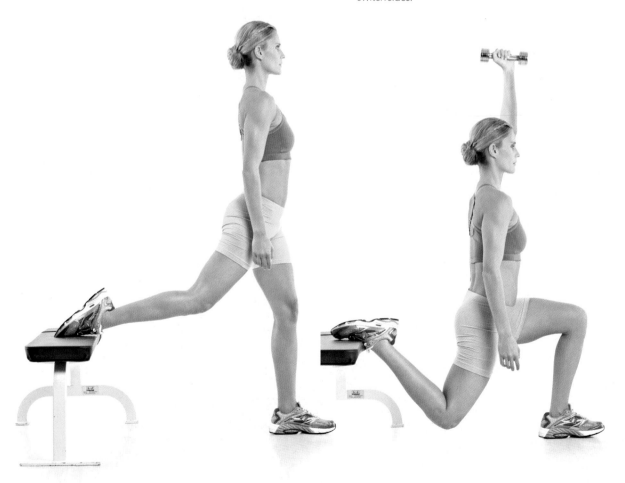

3B
wide-grip pulldown

start
* Sit at a pulldown machine—or, even better, do this kneeling in front of a pulley machine, as previously noted.

movement
* With your chest tall and stomach tight, grab the handles or bar with your palms facing away from you slightly wider than shoulder-width apart. Your arms should be fully extended. Pull the bar or handles down to gently touch your upper chest. Pause when you make contact, and then return to the start position and repeat.

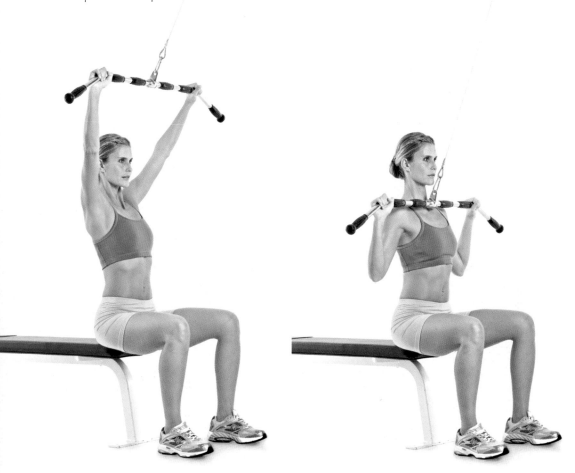

3C
single-leg, single-arm romanian deadlift

start

- Stand with a neutral spine and a dumbbell in your right hand using an overhand grip. Put all of your weight on your left leg. Raise your right foot slightly.

movement

- Push your hips back a few inches while keeping your back straight. Bend at the waist and lower the weight toward the floor as you maintain a neutral spine.

- As you descend, raise your right leg behind your body. You'll feel the stretch in your left hamstring. Go as low as you can while maintaining a neutral spine—try to touch the dumbbell to the floor, if you're able.

- Pause at the bottom and then slowly return to the starting position. Do all your reps and then repeat for the opposite side of your body. Add weight as you get stronger.

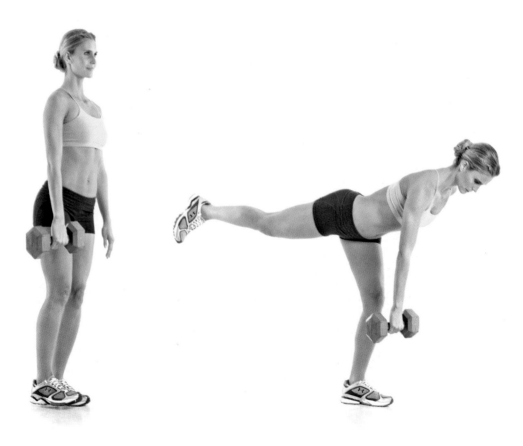

3D
inverted row

start

- Lie on your back on the floor under an Olympic bar that is placed securely in a squat rack just slightly beyond arm's length. Grab the bar with an overhand grip. Place your feet straight out in front of you and position the bar directly across from your chest. Lift your hips so your body is completely flat. The position should be like an upside-down pushup.

movement

- Performing a rowing motion, pull the upper body up to the bar so that the chest touches the bar. Keep your body completely flat through the entire motion.

Tip

If this position is too difficult, bend your knees and put your feet flat on the floor to decrease the load by putting more weight on your legs. Once the exercise becomes easy, raise your feet onto a bench, and eventually a Swiss ball.

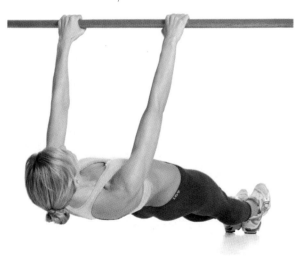
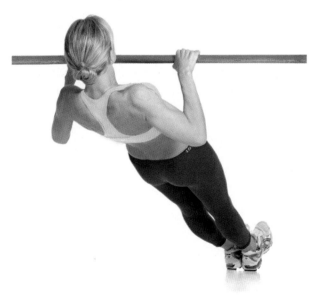

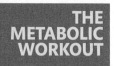

phase 3: WEEKS 7 TO 9

➽ In addition to your featherweight strength-training routine, you still need to do your interval workouts twice a week to experience the full results. Use the following exercises for Phase 3 and keep in mind that the scheduling flexibility of the previous phases applies here as well. If you want to continue the program after Week 9 and hone other troublesome spots, simply select one of the metabolic workouts you've already done, modify it according to the instructions below, and continue to do the workout twice a week.

1A Squat Thrust
1B Cross Behind Step Up and Over
1C Spiderman Pushup
1D Over/Under

instructions: Do each exercise as many times as you can for 60 seconds. Rest for 30 seconds and then advance to the next exercise. Complete 6 rounds total. Do not rest between rounds. These workouts should still be intense and short, but they'll take 36 minutes—12 more than you've been doing. Also, continue to add density every time you do the workout by trying to up your number of reps.

1A
squat thrust

start
• Stand with your feet slightly apart and your arms at your sides.

movement
• Quickly bend at your waist and touch the floor with your palms spread slightly wider than your shoulders.

• Putting weight on your hands, jump backward, extending your legs so you're in a pushup position.

• Pause for a moment, and then jump forward so that your feet are inside your hands again. Stand up, and repeat.

Tip
To make the exercise more advanced, jump into the air every time you're rising from the crouched position, and then return to the starting position.

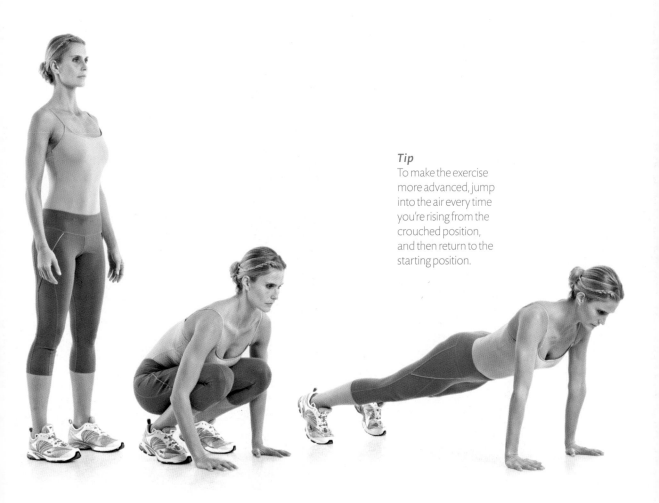

1B

cross behind step up and over

start

* Stand with a box (or bench) at your right side and place your right foot on the box.

movement

* Drive through your right leg and bring your left foot onto the box so that you're standing atop the box with both feet side by side.

* Keeping your right foot in the same position, cross your left leg behind you and place it on the opposite side of the box.

movement *(continued)*

* From there, drive through your right leg again to stand back up on the box, and then bring your left leg back down to end in the starting position. Do this for 30 seconds, then switch legs and repeat for another 30 seconds.

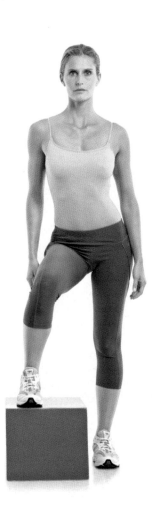
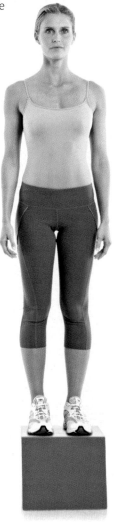
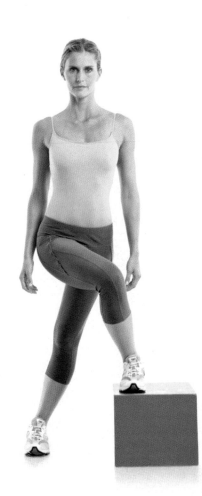

spider-man pushup

start

• Assume the standard pushup position.

movement:

• As you lower your body toward the floor, lift your right foot off the floor, swing your right leg out sideways, and try to touch your knee to your elbow, almost as if you were Spider-Man climbing a wall.

• Reverse the movement, then push your body back to the starting positon. Repeat, but on your next repetition, touch your left knee to your left elbow. Continue to alternate sides.

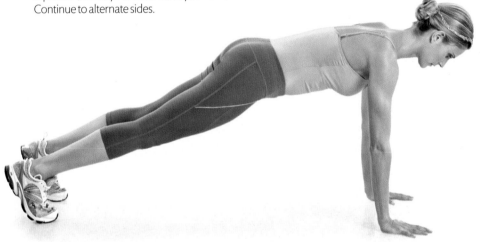

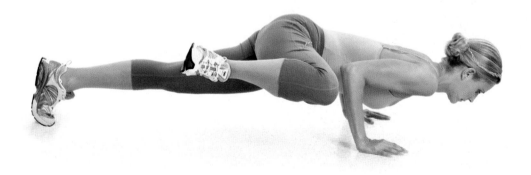

1D
over /under

start:

- Stand with your feet about shoulder-width apart. Imagine there's a stick at waist height on your right. You will first be stepping over the imaginary stick, and then ducking beneath it.

movement:

- Lift your left leg over the imaginary stick from left to right.

- Bring your left foot to the ground so that you're straddling the imaginary stick.

- Now lift your right foot off the ground, balance on your left leg, and bring your right foot up and over the stick.

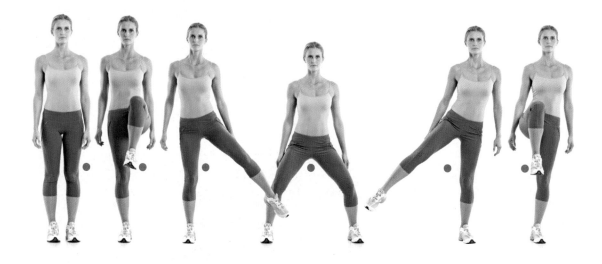

movement (*continued*)**:**

- You should now be standing in the original starting position with the imaginary stick to your right.

- Keeping your torso upright, duck into a squat so that your thighs are about parallel with the floor. Then step your right foot as far to your right as you can.

- Shifting your body weight from your left leg to your right, travel beneath the imaginary stick.

- You should now be in a squat position with your left foot extended. Bring it back beneath your hip, return to the starting position, and repeat the entire exercise.

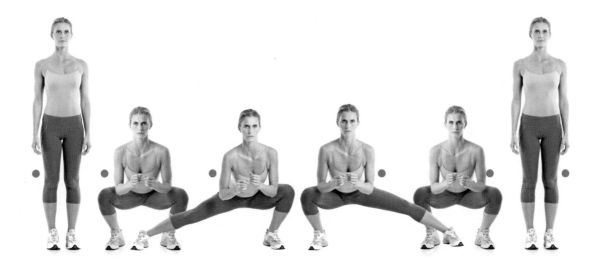

flat belly, thin waist

Whittle your middle and have a trim tummy forever

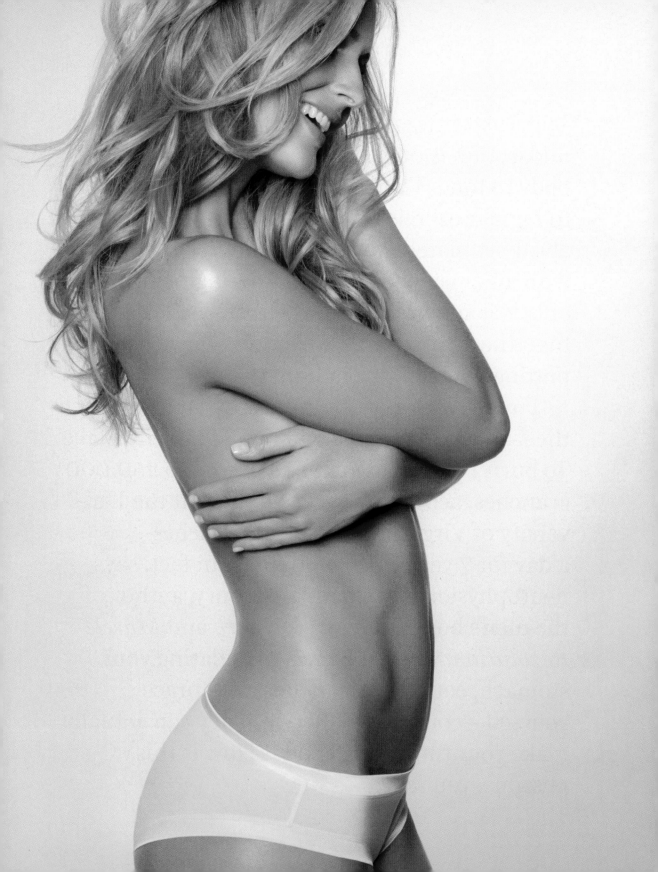

The frustrating reality is that for women, the midsection is one of the trickiest areas of the body to tone. That's why even those dedicated to regular exercise have trouble ironing out their abs. Fortunately, with expert help, I've come up with an amazing tummy-flattening plan. Not only is it supereffective; it's likely loads easier than the agonizing ab workouts you've been putting yourself through up to now.

I'm going to start by cutting straight through the fat: A ton of situps will not a flat belly make. To burn 1 pound of fat, you have to do 250,000 crunches, according to researchers at the University of Virginia. That's 100 crunches a day for 7 years. Uh, no thanks. In fact, says neurophysiologist Chad Waterbury, author of the men's books *Huge in a Hurry* and *Muscle Revolution,* when it comes to deflating your stomach, countless crunches are—brace yourself—counterproductive. They can actually make your tummy protrude! How is this possible, you ask?

Well, for one thing, the classic situp engages only the superficial abdominal muscles, those just under the skin—namely, the *rectus abdominis* (the muscle that, when developed correctly, comprises a "six-pack") and the *external obliques* (which are in the proximity of your love handles, if you have them). Now, even though these muscles are located in your abdomen instead of your arms, legs, or back, they share a similarity—namely, they're all made of muscle fibers. And just as countless biceps curls will result in larger biceps, countless situps will result in larger, not smaller, abs. Go ahead, let out a gasp. As I mentioned in Chapter 4, when you work a muscle, you cause microscopic tears in the fibers: The body repairs these tears by rebuilding the muscle, leaving it—eventually—slightly bigger than before. "Muscle tissue adapts to the demands placed on it," says Waterbury. "In general, when athletes want to pump up a muscle, they challenge it to a high volume of reps." So if you keep working and working your outer-layer abs, they're going to increase in size, and you'll wind up with—horror of all horrors— a *larger* belly and a poochier appearance. The effect will be even worse if you have a layer of fat on top of an overdeveloped abdomen, because the muscle will push the flab forward. Not so cute.

56% of women say that they'd like to permanently drop one to two sizes

To get a tighter, leaner tummy, you first have to target the muscles beneath the near-the-surface ones—namely, the *transversus abdominis*, the *multifidus*, and the *internal obliques*. These are the muscles that work together to hold in your torso and stabilize your spine. Strengthening them will pull in your middle like a corset (oh, if only Scarlett O'Hara had known!) and support your back (a boon if you've got chronic lower-back pain), which is why core-engaging fitness activities like yoga and Pilates work so well. In fact, researchers at Auburn University Montgomery in Alabama found that Pilates abdominal moves are superior to crunches for sculpting your midsection. Not only did the five exercises studied engage the deep-down ab muscles more fully than situps did, they also did a better job of tightening the external muscles. (Turn to page 140 to learn how to do them on your optional do-anything day.) What's more, exercising abdominal muscles *dynamically*—forcing them to contract over and over again as you lift your torso up and down—isn't as effective as targeting them *isometrically,* or holding the contraction without moving the muscle. With isometric exercises, says Waterbury, you'll strengthen the muscles but you'll also do considerably less damage to them, meaning you'll experience less muscle growth.

62%
of women say that the body part they're most self-conscious of is their belly!

Besides targeting the "hidden" muscles of your midsection, you also need to focus on your fanny. That's right: Your booty and your belly are partners in crime, according to LBN workout designer Rachel Cosgrove. Over time, sitting around too much renders your glutes practically useless and causes your hip flexors—the muscles that connect your hip bones to your legs—to become tight. This couch-potato combo tilts your pelvis forward, which increases the arch in your back and stresses your spine. "From a cosmetic standpoint," says Cosgrove, "it puts the bulge in your belly." So even if you've melted off every extra fat cell and strengthened your core muscles to the max, you'll *still* have some bulge to battle. To win that fight, you've got to both work your butt and loosen up your hip flexors.

But before we get into the specific moves that will bring your belly up to Look Better Naked snuff, I'd like to go over some of the other benefits of streamlining your midsection. Consider this bevy of payoffs:

Steamier Sex!

A smaller waistline means better blood flow. When you're overweight, you tend to have significantly more artery-clogging plaque, which decreases blood flow throughout the body. Researchers have found that increased blood flow in the pelvic region improves vaginal lubrication, sensitivity, arousal, and sensation.

Reduced Risk of Injury!

Researchers for the US Army tracked the injuries of male and female soldiers during a year of field training in which they periodically performed the standard army fitness test of situps, pushups, and a 2-mile run. Those who could crank out the most situps were less likely to suffer from injuries.

Improved Overall Health!

Studies show that people with flat abs are . . .
- 25% less likely to develop heart disease
- 35% less likely to have a heart attack
- 41% less likely to develop high blood pressure
- 40% less likely to develop kidney cancer
- 60% less likely to develop gallstones
- 14% less likely to develop osteoarthritis
- 63% less likely to develop asthma

A Longer Life!

A Canadian study of more than 8,000 people over a period of 13 years found that those with the weakest abs had more than double the death rate of folks with the strongest midsections.

Not a bad list of reasons to sculpt yourself some sexy abs—keep them in mind whenever your motivation wanes. The four exercises that comprise your customized ab circuit will help you achieve your flat-abs goal.

Just a few reminders before you start:

• *Engage your inner ab muscles.* Suck in your stomach as if you're anticipating being punched there, and maintain that braced-belly position for the duration of each exercise.

• *Tighten your glutes at the same time.* Squeezing your butt will also help support your lower back.

• *Keep your hips in a neutral position.* This will better enable you to strengthen your core.

CUSTOMIZED ABS WORKOUT

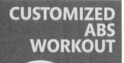

phase 3: WEEKS 7 TO 9

instructions: Perform 2 sets of 15 reps, resting 30 seconds between most exercises.

abs circuit

EXERCISE	SETS	REPS	TEMPO/TIME	REST
2A: Antirotation Reverse Lunge*	2	15/side	moderate	30 sec
2B: Side Plank	2	1/side	30 sec	30 sec
2C: Horizontal Wood Chop on Swiss Ball*	2	15/side	moderate	30 sec
2D: Hip Flexor Stretch	2	1/side	30 sec	30 sec

workout A

EXERCISES	SETS	REPS	TEMPO/TIME	REST
Dynamic Warmup	*See page 106*			
Circuit 1:				
1A: Plank on Swiss Ball	1-2	1	60–90 sec	60 sec
1B: Core Stability Twist	1-2	15	moderate	60 sec
Circuit 2:				
Customized abs circuit				
Circuit 3:				
3A: Hip Extension	2	15	moderate	30 sec
3B: One-Point Dumbbell Row*	2	15/side	moderate	30 sec
3C: Front Squat*	2	15	moderate	30 sec
3D: Single-Arm Dumbbell Chest Press on a Swiss Ball*	2	15/side	moderate	30 sec

workout B

EXERCISES	SETS	REPS	TEMPO/TIME	REST
Dynamic Warmup	*See page 106*			
Circuit 1:				
1A: Prone Jackknife	1-2	10–15/side	moderate	60 sec
1B: Prone Cobra on a Swiss Ball	1-2	1	60–90 sec	60 sec
Circuit 2:				
Customized abs circuit				
Circuit 3:				
3A: Split Squat with Opposite Arm Overhead Press*	2	15/side	moderate	30 sec
3B: Wide-Grip Pulldown*	2	15	moderate	30 sec
3C: Single-Leg, Single-Arm Romanian Deadlift*	2	15/side	moderate	30 sec
3D: Inverted Row	2	15	moderate	30 sec

* Add weight as you progress in the program.

2A

antirotation reverse lunge

start

• Stand with a pulley at shoulder height at your right side. Hold the pulley's handle with both hands and step away a few feet to create tension. Raise your arms so that they're straight out in front of you. Spread your feet about shoulder-width apart. You should feel your core engaged in order to hold your arms straight in front of you while resisting the tension from the pulley.

movement

• Keeping the tension on the pulley and your arms straight, step back with your right foot into a reverse lunge. Keep your core engaged and your chest tall. Return to the starting position and repeat.

• Do all your reps with one leg and then switch sides.

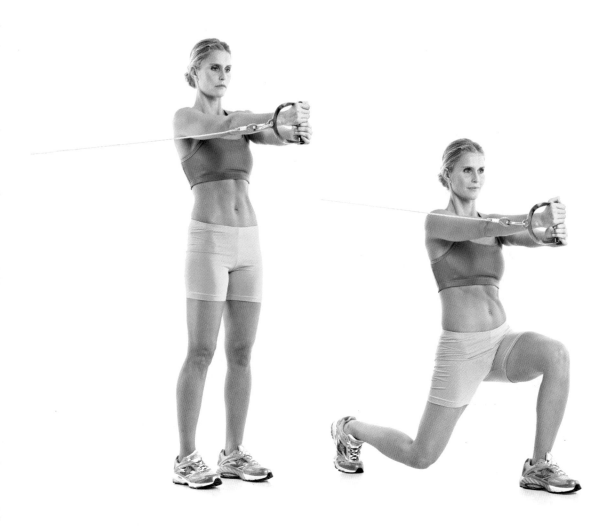

2B
side plank

Position

- Lie on your left side with your elbow underneath your shoulder. Your body should be in a straight line with your legs stacked one on top of the other. Balancing on your forearm and your foot, raise your hips as high as you can. Keep your core tight. Hold this position for the specified period of time, rest, and then switch sides.

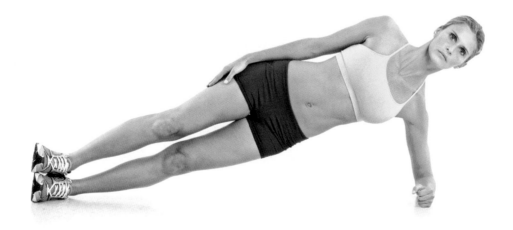

2C
horizontal wood chop on a swiss ball

start
- Position a Swiss ball alongside a pulley machine. Lower the pulley to the floor. With your back on the Swiss ball and your knees bent at a 90-degree angle, hold onto the handle with both hands and straight arms. Position your hands toward the pulley, and keep your eyes on them.

movement
- Keeping your arms straight and your eyes on your hands, pull the handle straight across your body until it's directly above your head. Return to the start under control and repeat. Do all your reps for one side and then switch sides.

Tip
If using a Swiss ball is too difficult, you can also do this exercise standing up.

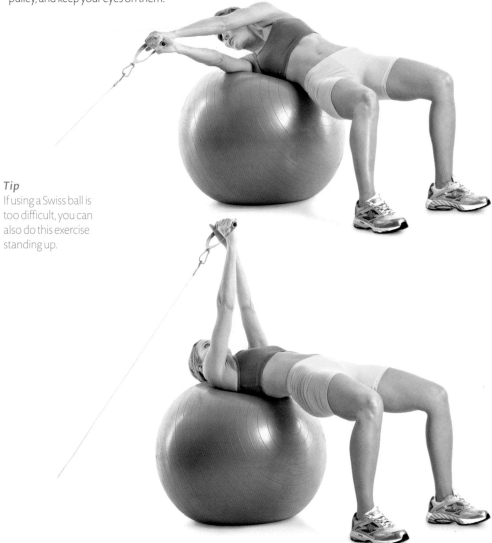

hip-flexor stretch
,2D

start

- Kneel on your right knee, your left foot flat on the floor. Keep your torso upright and rest your hands on your left knee.

movement

- Gently push your hips forward while keeping your torso upright. You should feel a stretch in the front of your right hip. Hold the stretch for 60 seconds, switch legs, and repeat.

- To intensify the stretch, turn your body away from your back leg. You can also raise your right arm straight over your head and lean away from your back leg.

Tip

For a different version of this exercise, stand facing away from a bench. Place your right foot on the bench and lower into a lunge, as if you were doing a split squat (see page 155), but then lean forward to feel the stretch in the front of your hip.

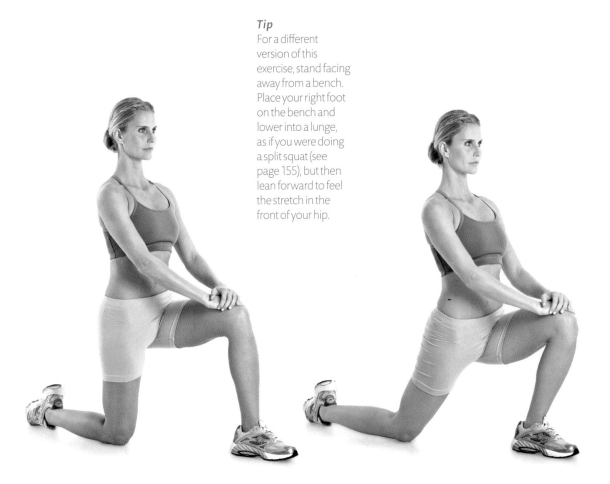

eat, drink, and still *shrink*

➤ You can't see the results of your belly-flattening efforts if they're hidden under a layer of fat. Fortunately, there are plenty of proven strategies for melting off excess ab flab. These are the most effective ones—all of which you've been doing as part of the LBN diet.

• Eliminate Added Sugar

The average American eats about 20 teaspoons of sugar each day in the form of processed foods such as soda, baked goods, breakfast cereals, fruit drinks, and even flavored yogurt—about 325 empty calories' worth! Plus, all that sugar increases insulin production, which slows metabolism.

• Pump Up Your Protein Intake

Substituting meat, fish, dairy, and nuts for carbohydrates can reduce the amount of fat around your middle. Researchers at McMaster University in Canada assessed the diets of 617 people and discovered that when they switched out carbs in favor of an equal amount of protein, they reduced overall belly fat.

• Order Smart at Happy Hour

Replace your calorie-packed margarita with my Look Better Naked cocktail or a glass of wine. Research shows that beer drinkers, in particular, have the most belly fat. And then pace yourself: A study from the University of Buffalo found that binge drinkers (people who typically down more than three or four drinks at a time) have more ab fat than people who sip the same quantity of alcohol over several days.

• Don't Fear Fat

Research shows that diets containing more than 50 percent fat are just as effective for weight loss as those that are low in fat. "Fat is filling and adds flavor to food—both of which help prevent you from feeling deprived, so you'll be less likely to overeat," says Alan Aragon, MS, a nutritionist in the Los Angeles area. Eat foods rich in monounsaturated fats, aka MUFAs, the celebrated belly fat-targeting foods; research has even found that it's okay to enjoy whole foods that contain saturated fat (including milk, cheese, and butter) in moderation.

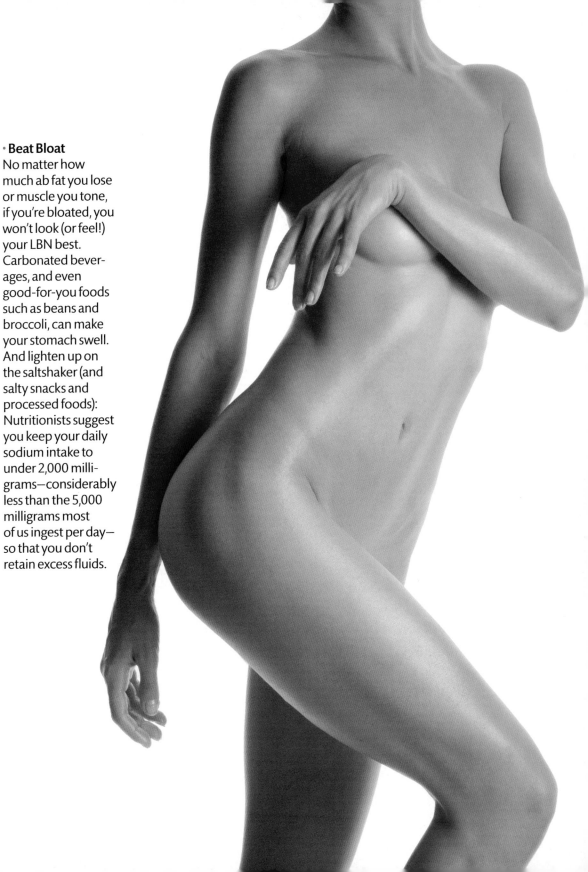

• Beat Bloat
No matter how much ab fat you lose or muscle you tone, if you're bloated, you won't look (or feel!) your LBN best. Carbonated beverages, and even good-for-you foods such as beans and broccoli, can make your stomach swell. And lighten up on the saltshaker (and salty snacks and processed foods): Nutritionists suggest you keep your daily sodium intake to under 2,000 milligrams—considerably less than the 5,000 milligrams most of us ingest per day—so that you don't retain excess fluids.

Control
Your Cravings...

...and stop them from sabotaging your abs in a moment of weakness

➡ Absolutely nobody likes a nag. But try telling that to the bag of snack-size Snickers bars that won't stop calling your name, or the oh-so-salty french fries that keep pummeling your willpower.

A craving is like a little devil, constantly encouraging you to indulge. Dieting turns up the pressure, and we all know that giving in to urges is a ticket to nothing-in-my-closet-fits hell.

The good news is that unlike, say, your mom's constant probing about future grandkids, these unhealthy tormentors can be fended off. The reason: Cravings are all about blood sugar. If your levels stay consistent throughout the day, your eating patterns will too. It's when you starve yourself for hours that cravings call. "Your blood sugar can fall too low after just 4 hours of not eating," says Valerie Berkowitz, MS, RD, director of nutrition at the Center for Balanced Health in New York City. So you search the fridge, the food court, even the seat cushions for simple carbohydrates that will give you a quick boost.

Trouble is, the resulting blood sugar spike triggers your pancreas to release insulin, a hormone that not only lowers blood sugar but also signals your body to run through the craving cycle over and over. In about half of us, insulin tends to overshoot—that's what sends blood sugar crashing. "This reinforces the binge because it makes you crave sugar and starch again," Berkowitz says. In other words, giving in to a carb craving

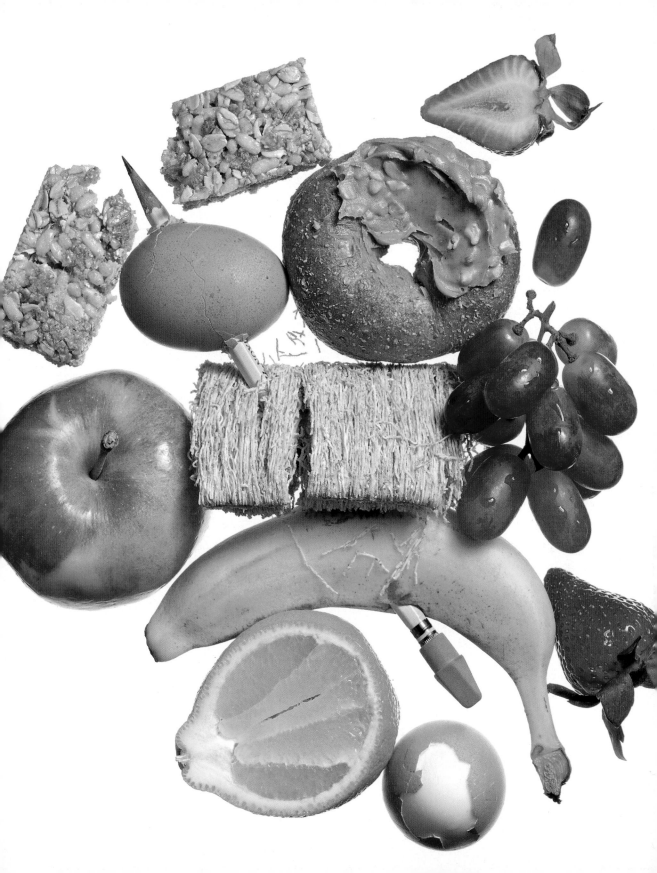

only leaves you wanting more. So how do you prevent yourself from reaching for that candy bar? By following these seven steps designed to stop 99 percent of cravings before they start—and to help you muzzle the 1 percent that never seem to shut up.

1. Ramp Up Your Resolve

One reason most diets fail is that long-term goals can be deceptively difficult: When the plan is to watch what you eat for the next 6 months, chugging one caramel latte with whipped cream seems like a minor slip. To avoid that kind of thinking, commit to eating well for a fixed amount of time that you're 100 percent confident you can manage, even if it's just a few days. "Once you make it to your goal date, start over," says Mary Vernon, MD, chairwoman of the board of the American Society of Bariatric Physicians. "This establishes the notion that you can be successful and gives you a chance to notice that eating better makes you feel better, reinforcing your desire to continue."

2. Find Meaningful Motivation

Yes, you're aiming to look better naked, but that doesn't mean you can't simultaneously be striving for some deeper benefits. "Arm yourself with additional motivators," says Jeff Volek, PhD, RD, an associate professor of kinesiology at the University of Connecticut in Storrs. Keep a daily journal in which you monitor headaches, heartburn, acne, canker sores, and sleep quality. "Discovering that your new diet improves the quality of your life and health is powerful motivation," Volek says.

3. Move On After a Mistake

Okay, you overindulged. Now what? "Forget about it," says James Newman, a nutritionist at Tahlequah City Hospital in Oklahoma, who followed his own advice to shed 300 pounds. "Don't assume that you've failed or fallen off the wagon." Institute a simple rule: Follow any "cheat" meal with at least five healthy meals and snacks.

13 Flat-Belly Food Tricks

Simple shortcuts that will help you slim down

1. Eat Dessert
Yes, always. "A small amount can signal that the meal is over," says Barbara Rolls, PhD, author of The Volumetrics Eating Plan. She ends her meals with a piece of high-quality chocolate.

2. Get a Mustache
Consuming 1,800 milligrams of calcium a day could block the absorption of about 80 calories, according to a University of Tennessee study. Jump-start your calcium intake by filling your coffee mug with fat-free or 1 percent milk, drinking it down to the level you want in your coffee, then pouring in your caffeine fix. That's 300 milligrams down, 1,500 to go.

3. Spice Things Up
Capsaicin, the substance that puts the hot in hot pepper, temporarily boosts your metabolism. Dairy blocks capsaicin's sweat-inducing signals better than water, though, so pair it with your favorite searing-hot dishes.

4. Go Organic
That's where you're likely to find bread and cereal with fiber counts that put the conventional choices to shame. Thought you were doing well with your 3-grams-per-serving Cheerios? Nature's Path Optimum Slim blows it away with 9 grams.

5. Keep the Skin On
Speaking of fiber, a lot of it's in the peel, whether it's potatoes, apples, or pears. Even oranges: Don't eat the whole peel, but keep the pith, that white, stringy stuff—it's packed with heart-healthy compounds called flavonoids.

6. Buy Precut Vegetables
Sure, they cost more, but you're more likely to eat them. "Make low-energy snacks as easy as possible," Rolls says. "Keep vegetables as near to hand as you can. Make it so you have no excuse."

7. Use Zagat's
Pick restaurants where you'll actually want to linger. "When the meals are not hurried, you can regulate your attitude," says Roberta Anding, a spokeswoman for the American Dietetic Association. That means your body—not the empty plate—will tell you when to stop.

8. Always Snack at 3 p.m.
"Having a low-calorie snack [now] can stave off cravings for high-cal foods that might crop up later," Anding says. An ounce of nuts or two sticks of string cheese weigh in at about 170 calories.

9. Drink with Your Dominant Hand
If you're circulating at a party, Rolls suggests keeping your glass in the hand you eat with. If you're drinking with it, you can't eat with it.

10. Plate It
Whatever it is, don't eat it out of the container and don't bring the container to the couch. "Part of satiety is visual," Anding says. "Your brain actually has to see the food on the plate, and when you reach into the jar or the box or the bag, you don't see it." If it's worth eating, put it on a plate.

Eat what's there, then stop.

11. Start with Salad
It's the holy grail of dieting—eat less by eating more. Rolls' research has found that eating a salad as a first course decreased total lunch calories by 12 percent. Avoid the croutons and creamy dressings, which have the opposite effect.

12. Go Public
Enlist the help of friends, family, and co-workers—and know they're watching. "The power of embarrassment is greater than willpower," says Stephen Gullo, PhD, author of The Thin Commandments.

13. Use Your Fingers
Find a way other than food to work off your nervous energy. "It's behavior modification," Anding says. "Instead of grabbing chips, you pick up your knitting—or anything else that occupies your hands."

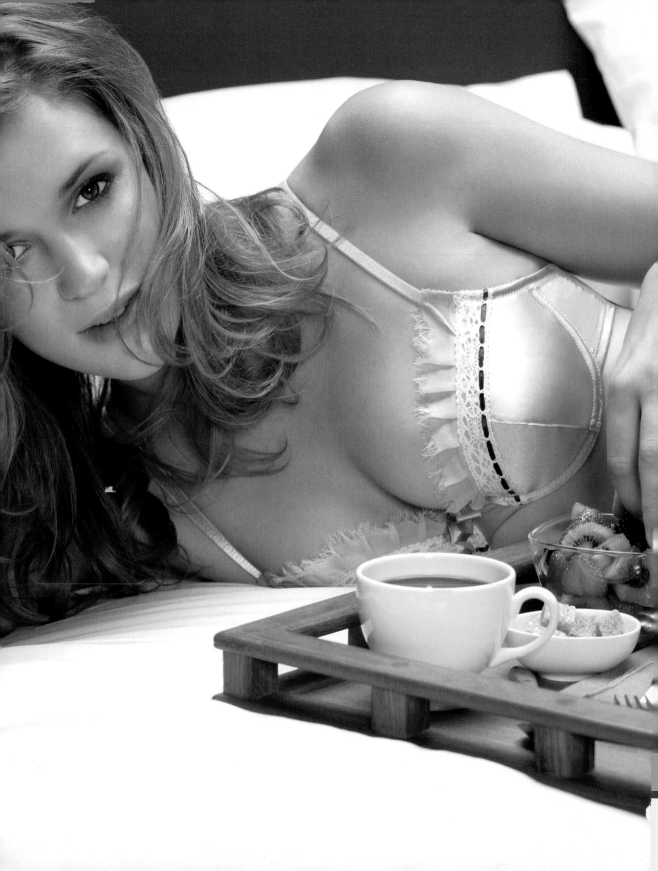

4. Roll Out of Bed and Into the Kitchen

If you sleep for 6 to 8 hours and then skip breakfast, your body is essentially running on fumes by the time you get to work. And that sends you desperately seeking sugar, which is exactly what you don't want to find.

5. Restock Your Shelves

You're more likely to give in to a craving when the object you desire is close at hand. So make sure it's not: Toss the junk food and restock your cupboard, fridge, and workspace with almonds and other nuts, low-fat cheeses, fruits and vegetables, and canned tuna and salmon.

6. Think Like a Biochemist

Cookies made with organic cane juice might sound like something your yoga teacher would eat, but they won't help her fit into her Lycra pants. Junk food by any other name is still junk. Ditto for lots of "health foods" in the granola aisle. "Natural" sweeteners such as honey raise blood sugar just like the white stuff. "If you're going to eat cookies, accept that you're deviating from your plan, and then revert to your diet afterward," Berkowitz says. Kidding yourself will only get you in trouble.

7. Spot Hunger Impostors

Have a craving for sweets even though you ate just an hour ago? Imagine sitting down to a meal, instead. "If you're truly hungry, the steak will sound good, and you should eat," says Richard Feinman, PhD, a professor of biochemistry at the State University of New York Downstate Medical Center in Brooklyn. "If it doesn't sound good, your brain is playing tricks on you." His advice: Distract yourself, which can be as easy as stretching at your desk or turning your attention to a different task. Also, thirst often masquerades as hunger, so as silly as it sounds, drink a glass of water and see if that quells the pang for munchies.

firm chest, beautiful breasts

Exercises—plus beauty and bedroom
tricks—that target your twins

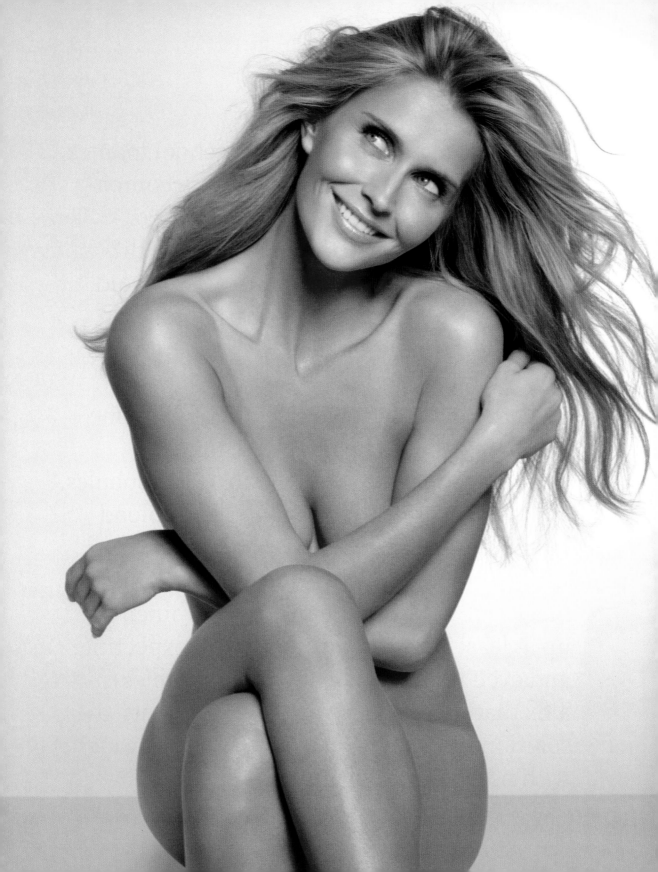

"We must, we must, we must increase our bust!" Remember that middle-school mantra, and the ridiculous "exercise" that accompanied it—elbows bent like chicken wings, pumping back and forth, back and forth? Lot of good that did any of our 13-year-old chests: We all got what Mother Nature intended, whether it was a perky petite pair or a full buxom set.

That's because, of course, there's not one iota of muscle tissue in human breasts. They're made up of fat, milk ducts and lobules, connective tissue, lymph nodes, and blood vessels—none of which respond to being "trained." The only ways to make your breasts bigger are to get pregnant (most women go up at least a cup size when they're expecting, and even more if they nurse their babies), a fix that's temporary; or to get implants, a solution that can be permanent but is fraught with potential problems.

I don't mean to deflate your hopes of enhancing your chest. Even though you can't increase the size of your breasts themselves, you *can* make them more attractive. For starters, you can develop the muscles that lie behind your ladies—your pectoralis major and minor—with pressing exercises. There's just one caveat: "You have to balance the presses with rowing exercises that strengthen your mid-back. If you don't, you'll develop a forward posture that will make your boobs look droopy," explains LBN workout designer Rachel Cosgrove.

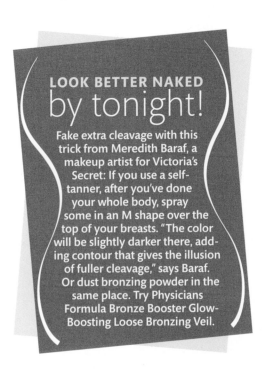

LOOK BETTER NAKED
by tonight!

Fake extra cleavage with this trick from Meredith Baraf, a makeup artist for Victoria's Secret: If you use a self-tanner, after you've done your whole body, spray some in an M shape over the top of your breasts. "The color will be slightly darker there, adding contour that gives the illusion of fuller cleavage," says Baraf. Or dust bronzing powder in the same place. Try Physicians Formula Bronze Booster Glow-Boosting Loose Bronzing Veil.

For that reason, the primary goal of this workout has less to do with what's up front than what's in back: "When you stand up straight and pull your shoulders back, your breasts immediately perk up," says Cosgrove. So here you'll find moves that will strengthen your back and shoulder muscles, as well as your core. If your torso is strong, solid, and erect, your breasts will have a nice "shelf" to sit atop. In addition to the muscle-building moves, there's a stretch for your chest muscles that will allow them to work through a full range of motion.

Before we get to work, let's go over an important fringe benefit of this routine—namely, the improvement it will make to your posture.

Maybe your stance isn't a priority when you hit the gym—good posture, like the instructions that came with your cell phone, usually gets filed away in a bottom drawer somewhere. But it's something worth thinking about, whether you're standing in a line, sitting on a couch, or, worst of all, working at a desk. Why is that last one so problematic? The average human head

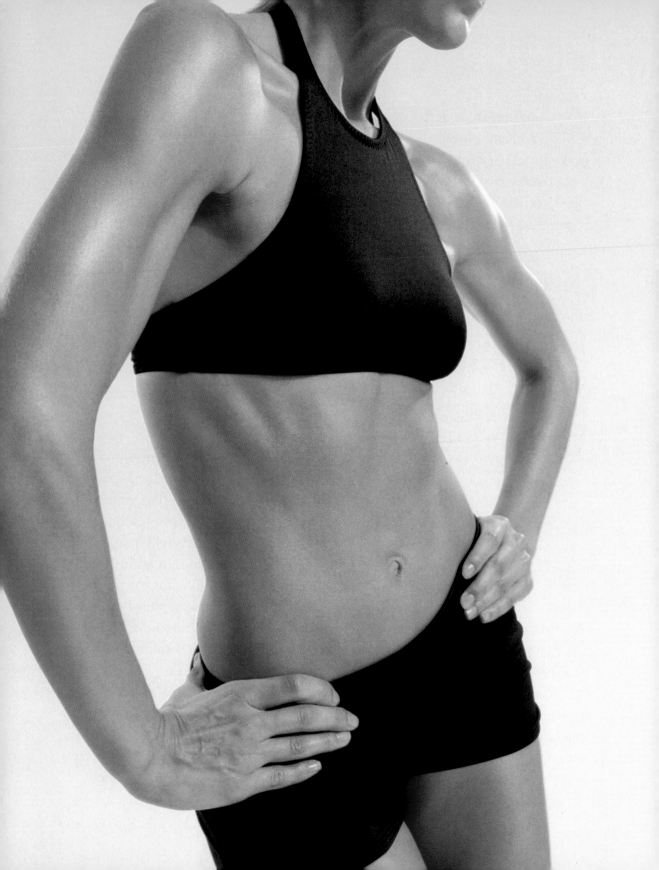

weighs 8 pounds. If your chin drifts forward just 3 inches—as it tends to when you stare at a computer—the muscles of your neck, shoulders, and upper back must support the equivalent of 11 pounds. That's a weight-bearing increase of 38 percent, often for hours at a time, and your body compensates by letting you slouch forward and round your shoulders. If you're not careful, that becomes a permanent adjustment.

Not only does good posture make you look taller and slimmer, it also improves your energy and digestion. "When you slouch, less oxygen makes it to your muscles, and the bloodflow to your gut is impaired, causing indigestion. You also get headaches from cramped neck muscles and, frankly, look lousy," says chiropractor Drew DeMann of Manhattan Spine and Sports Medicine. The spine is your body's shock absorber; let-

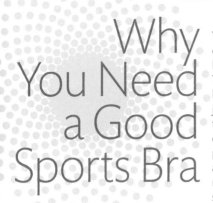

Why You Need a Good Sports Bra

Your breasts are attached to your chest by a network of thin, delicate bands called Cooper's ligaments. They're designed to keep your breasts standing at attention, but, just like rubber bands, they lose their elasticity over time, and become increasingly slack. In large part this loosening is a function of age, but intense bouncing and movement can exacerbate it. Researchers at the University of Portsmouth, England, found that breasts can fly as much as 8 inches up and down regardless of size. They also go in and out and left to right in a sort of figure-eight pattern. The result: prematurely drooping grandma boobs.

Because you can't rebuild ligaments the way you can increase muscle mass, exercise will not reverse the damage once the sag has set in, so it's essential to shell out for a well-constructed, properly fitting, supportive sports bra. Look for one that encapsulates each breast in a separate chamber (rather than a shelf style), in a high-performance fabric that wicks away sweat, such as CoolMax or Double Dry. Look for styles that are sized according to cup (rather than those labeled "small," "medium," or "large." Once you find your dream bra, take good care of that baby. The chemicals in sweat break down Lycra, making it less supportive. Handwash your bra in cool water with a mild soap like Forever New (forevernew.com) or Ivory Snow after every workout. If you do toss it into a machine, use the gentle cycle and enclose it in a net bag with the bra's hooks fastened. To dry, always hang it up or lay it flat; dryers ruin elastic.

ting it slump causes imbalances, forcing the muscles and ligaments in your neck, shoulders, back, and legs to compensate.

Hunching can also affect your health: A 2007 study done at the University of Leeds in England found a link between muscles in the neck and a part of the brain stem that regulates blood pressure and heart rate. There's more: Rounding your back presses the rib cage and internal organs against your lungs, keeping them from expanding efficiently. The result: Less oxygen gets to your muscles. None of which, of course, will help your boobs look better. Whether your goal is to prive your pair or to look and feel better all over, here's a 3-week plan that will help you achieve your goals.

CUSTOMIZED BREAST WORKOUT

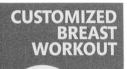

phase 3: WEEKS 7 TO 9

instructions: Perform 2-3 sets of 10 reps, resting 30 seconds between most exercises.

breast circuit

EXERCISE	SETS	REPS	TEMPO/TIME	REST
2A: Pushup-Position Row*	2-3	10/side	moderate	30 sec
2B: Alternating Incline Dumbbell Chest Press*	2-3	10/side	moderate	30 sec
2C: Standing Split-Stance Single-Arm Cable Row*	2-3	10/side	moderate	30 sec
2D: Chest Stretch	2-3	1/side	30 sec	30 sec

workout A

EXERCISES	SETS	REPS	TEMPO/TIME	REST
Dynamic Warmup	See page 106			
Circuit 1:				
1A: Plank on Swiss Ball	1-2	1	60–90 sec	60 sec
1B: Core Stability Twist	1-2	15/side	moderate	60 sec
Circuit 2:				
Customized Breast Circuit				
Circuit 3:				
3A: Hip Extension	2-3	10	moderate	30 sec
3B: One-Point Dumbbell Row*	2-3	10/side	moderate	30 sec
3C: Front Squat*	2-3	10	moderate	30 sec
3D: Single-Arm Dumbbell Chest Press on a Swiss Ball*	2-3	10/side	moderate	30 sec

workout B

EXERCISES	SETS	REPS	TEMPO/TIME	REST
Dynamic Warmup	See page 106			
Circuit 1:				
1A: Prone Jackknife	1-2	10–15/side	moderate	60 sec
1B: Prone Cobra on a Swiss Ball	1-2	1	60–90 sec	60 sec
Circuit 2:				
Customized Breast Circuit				
Circuit 3:				
3A: Split Squat with Opposite Arm Overhead Press*	2-3	10/side	moderate	30 sec
3B: Wide-Grip Pulldown*	2-3	10	moderate	30 sec
3C: Single-Leg, Single-Arm Romanian Deadlift*	2-3	10/side	moderate	30 sec
3D: Inverted Row	2-3	10	moderate	30 sec

*Add weight as you progress in the program.

2A
pushup-position row

start

- Get into a pushup position, with a dumbbell in each hand. (Hexagonal dumbbells work best, as their sides provide a sturdy base.)

movement

- Keep your body in a straight line while you lower yourself toward the floor to do a pushup (not pictured).

- As you return to the starting position, pull the dumbbell in your right hand from the floor in a rowing motion until it reaches your torso.

- Return the weight to the floor, do another pushup, and then do a row with your left arm. Continue to alternate arms for the designated number of reps.

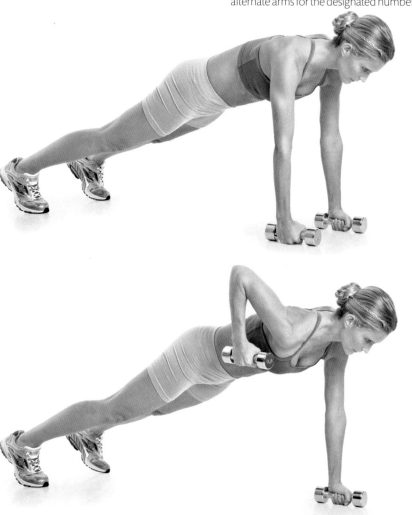

2B
alternating incline dumbbell chest press

start
- Lie on a Swiss ball with your hips unsupported, which will force you to contract your butt and leg muscles.

- Hold a dumbbell in each hand alongside your breasts. Push them straight up, keeping your core flexed as you do so.

movement
- Lower the right dumbbell until it's even with your breast.

- Perform a chest press to bring it back alongside the other dumbbell, and then switch and repeat with your left arm.

Tip
You can also do this on a Bosu ball or at the edge of a bench with your hips off the edge and just your upper back supported.

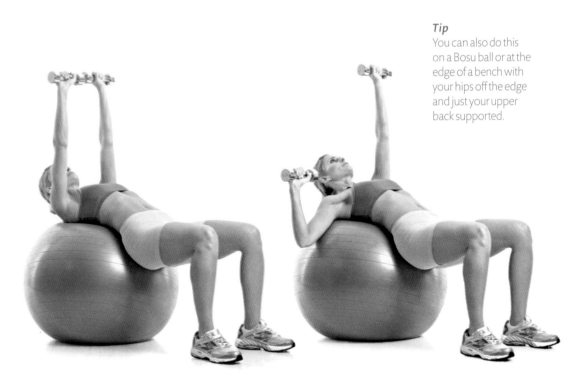

2C
split-stance single-arm cable row

start

• Face a high cable pulley with a handle attached. Stand in a split stance with your left foot in front of your right. Grasp the handle with your right hand. Position your body so that your arm is fully extended at shoulder height and the desired weight is barely separated from the rest of the stack.

movement

• Keeping your elbow close to your body and your shoulders down, pull the cable to the right side of your right breast, use your back muscles to squeeze your shoulder blades together.

• Pause, and then slowly extend your arm to the starting position, resisting the load along the way. Repeat for the designated repetitions and then switch arms.

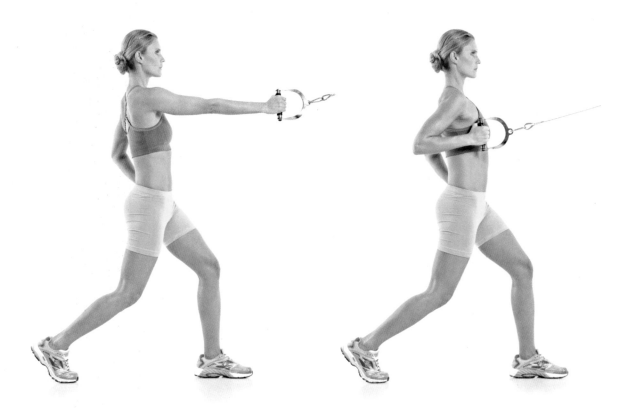

2D
chest stretch

position
- With your right palm and forearm firmly against a wall or doorway and your elbow at a 90-degree angle, walk or lean your torso forward to stretch your chest. Repeat on the opposite side.

Tip
For an alternate version, lie on a foam roller, positioned so that it's beneath your spine and also supports your head. Relax your arms at your sides until you begin to feel a stretch in your chest. Bend your elbows at a 90-degree angle and try raising them slightly to increase the stretch even more.

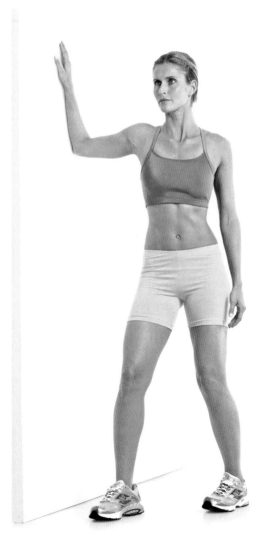

get 'em high

(With a Little Help from Your Man)

➥ What's the number-one reason you want to look better naked? I'm going to venture that it's got something to do with your favorite guy. If that's the case, then I would be remiss if I overlooked that reason in this particular chapter, given the huge role that breasts play in bed—or should play. Because if you feel so self-conscious about your chest that, even in the heat of the moment, you're not excited to remove your top, you're missing out on a prime source of satisfaction for you both. Not only that, but—and here's why I'm even going there in a book about improving your appearance—letting your breasts in on the fun will make 'em look better. First off, they'll double your pleasure at the very least, and a happy body is a sexy body. What most women don't realize is that their boobs can give them heaps of satisfaction. "The majority of research is geared toward keeping breasts healthy, and not nearly enough is known about how women can enjoy their breasts during sex," says Debby Herbenick, PhD, a sexual-health educator at the Kinsey Institute at Indiana University. Here's what researchers do know—and how you can use their discoveries to your personal LBN advantage.

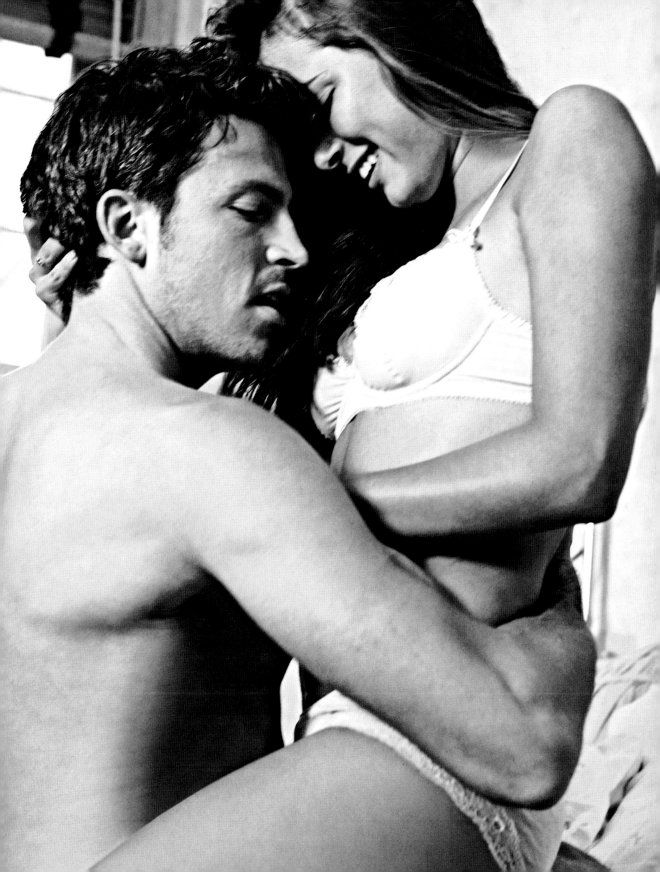

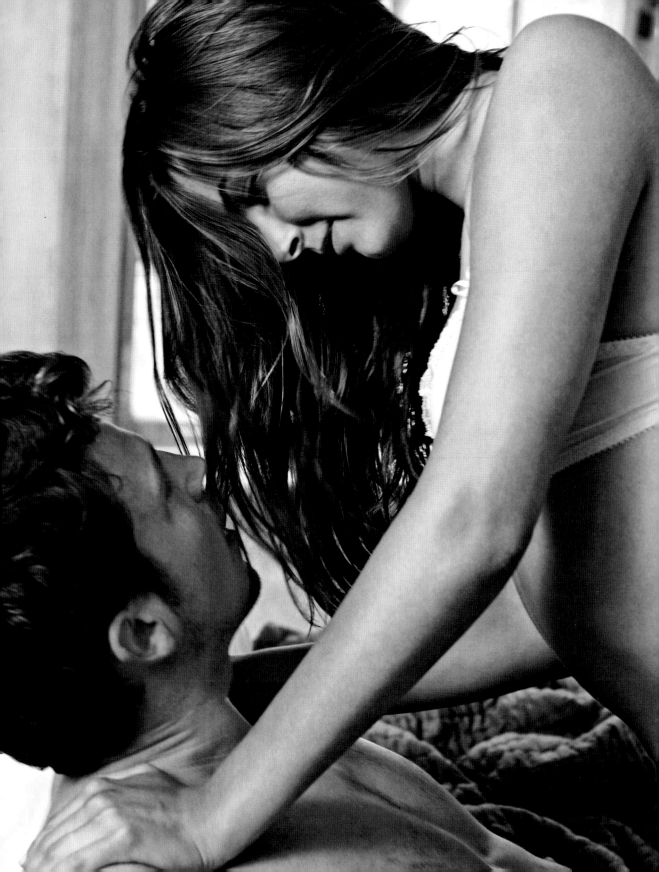

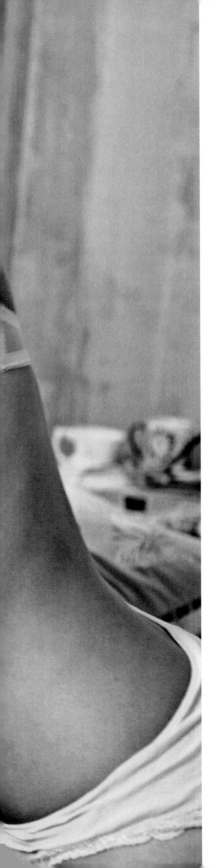

Supersizer

Your breasts may be his go-to spot on your bod, but how often do you luxuriate in the sensuality of your own curves? Never? Well, you're missing out. "Some women don't take the opportunity to relish their breasts during sex, especially if they're self-conscious about their cup size," says Ian Kerner, PhD, author of *She Comes First.* But guess what—all women, regardless of bra size, have the same number of nerve endings. If you'd like to head to bed in all your glory, spend a little time alone caressing yourself, thinking about the fun to come, your guy's gorgeous body—whatever it takes to get you in the mood. The LBN payoff of this self-indulgence? Experts say that breasts can grow up to 25 percent bigger when aroused.

Instant Perk-O-Lator

The same way a guy can become erect just-like-that, a woman's breasts can stand at attention sans direct contact. In fact, the mere suggestion of sexual touch can fire off pleasurable sensations in your breasts. To make your hills come alive without actually touching them, "have your guy rest his fingertips lightly on your sternum (the middle of your chest), then move them toward either breast, drawing light circles over the entire area," says Jaiya, co-author of *Red Hot Touch.*

Nip Untuck

Those nipples, they're always hogging the spotlight. But they're actually not the most sensitive regions of the chest. The flesh directly above the areola (the colored skin surrounding the nipple) is the real star of the show. "We think of nipples as primary erogenous zones—which they are, to a degree—but that's partially because they're so visible," Jaiya says. "However, studies have shown that women feel more pleasurable sensations above them." Have your guy rub the 10 o'clock–to–2 o'clock zones with an ice cube, then blow hot air on the wet parts for head-to-toe chills. Or he can use the tip of his tongue to lick circles around the area, slowly moving down to your nipple and areola (the second-most sensitive zone on your breast). The pressure from his tongue will activate a tiny muscle just beneath the surface that will, uh, flip on your headlights.

Get Straight

Halt your hunch

Pilates

Two prereqs for any Pilates move: First, engage your inner abs, which support the muscles in your back, and second, lift and lengthen your upper body. "Think of your spine as a bendy straw," says New York City Pilates instructor Kristin McGee. Everyday movements such as walking, sitting, and driving compact that straw. Pilates stretches it out again. "People say they grow an inch in class," McGee says. "It's really just that you find the space in your spine that you always had."

Try it: *The X*
Lie on your stomach with your arms and legs extended, forming an X. Brace your abs and relax your shoulders. Inhale and lift your arms and legs off the floor, making sure your legs go no higher than your arms. Exhale, bending your elbows toward your waist and pulling your legs together. Repeat 6 to 8 times.

Ballet

There's a reason you can spot a ballet dancer when she's not in her tutu: She's the one with the stick-straight posture. "Much of ballet is designed to lengthen the body from the base of the spine to the crown of the head," says Elise Gulan, a former professional dancer and the creator of the DVD *Element: Ballet Conditioning*. "Ballerinas are taught to pull their abs in and up. Doing so creates a lift in the spine." Take this cue: Imagine you have a string tied to the top of your head and somebody is pulling it from above.

Try it: *Port de Bras*
Stand with your heels touching and your toes turned out. Brace your abs. Keeping your shoulders down, raise both arms overhead. Bend forward, reaching your hands toward your toes while keeping your back flat. Go only as far as you can without losing your form. Brace your abs again, stand up, and, with arms still raised, arch backward slightly. Repeat 8 times.

Yoga

The spine is responsible for sending messages throughout your body, and when you're hunched, the pathway isn't as smooth, says Alison West, co-director of Yoga Union Center for Backcare and Scoliosis in New York City. Yoga strengthens the muscles that extend and realign your spine so your vertebrae aren't squished.

Try it: *Extended Side-Angle Pose*
Stand with your feet about 4 feet apart and turn your left foot out about 90 degrees. Extend your arms, palms down, at shoulder height. Bend your left knee until it's over your ankle. Flex from the waist to the left and place your left hand outside your left foot. (If you can't reach the floor, place your elbow or your hand on the inside of your knee instead.) Reach your right arm over your ear and turn your chin toward your right armpit. Look up and take five slow breaths. Return to standing, then switch sides. Repeat 3 to 5 times. New to yoga? Do the move with your back against a wall, so that you can concentrate on lengthening your spine and rolling your chest open.

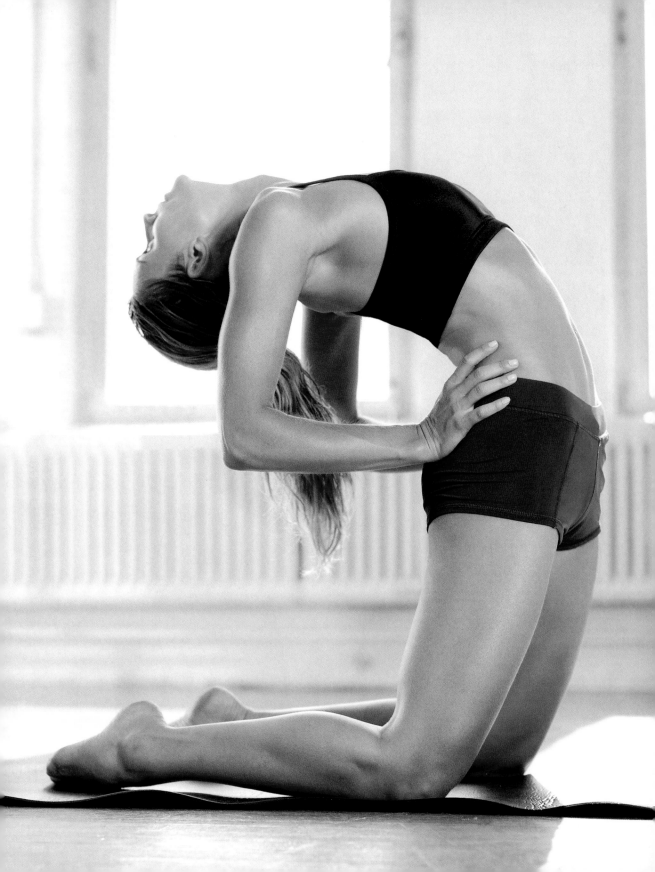

lean legs, tight butt

A fail-proof strategy for a dimple-free lower half

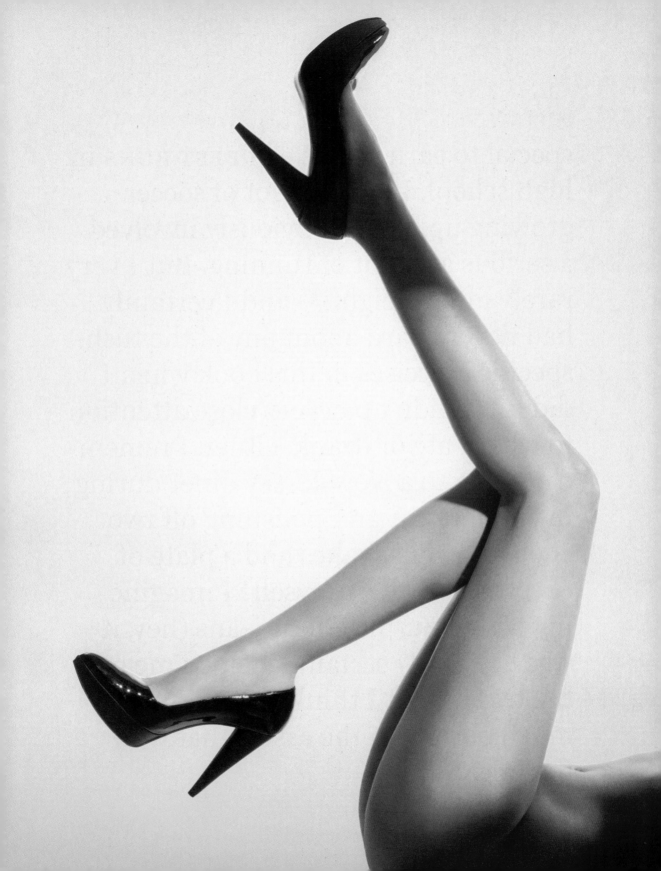

A confession: I didn't do anything special to earn the title of BEST BUNS in high school. I played a lot of soccer growing up, which obviously involved a serious amount of running. But I very rarely lifted weights—and I certainly had never heard about any of the tush-specific exercises in this book when I did lift. I didn't pay very close attention to what I ate or drank, either. I remember going to a New Jersey diner during my junior year and polishing off two chocolate milkshakes and a plate of cheese fries, all by myself! I imagine my prized purple Guess jeans (hey, it was the '80s!) certainly helped me bag the trophy, but I think I was pretty much born with the assets that won that award.

Oh, to be 17 years old again!

But anyone beyond the high school years knows that acquiring an admirable derriere is no easy feat. Our glutes—despite being the largest and one of the most powerful muscles in our bodies—can be difficult muscles to target. "We're much more reliant on our quadriceps," says Mike Mejia, a strength and conditioning specialist in Long Island, New York. "Most of us use them for everything. Next time you're walking up stairs or getting out of a chair, notice how much you rely on your thighs."

As a result, our bums get the short shrift. Without regular maintenance, they'll start to flatten out like a pancake or get saggy. Jeans can only disguise those unfortunate realities. The permanent solution requires you to get up off your butt and use it! Compound moves such as the stepups, squats, and deadlifts that make up the lower-body segment of this LBN workout are the most efficient way to zero in on your neglected "posterior chain," which is made up of the muscles you otherwise know as glutes, hamstrings, calves, and erector spinae. These muscles run the whole length of the back side of your body and they work together as a unit. Weaknesses here can often manifest themselves elsewhere, causing pain and injuries in seemingly unrelated locations, such as your knees and back. But by treating them like the team that they are, you'll strengthen and tone the main event—your butt—by giving it more lift and shape. Of course, the effect will be even greater if you're simultaneously eliminating fat. Your newly honed moon is surely going to shine!

LOOK BETTER NAKED by tonight!

Fake sleeker legs with a bronzer stick like Tarte Glam Gams Leg Bronzing Stick ($30, sephora.com). Just rub it down the center of your thighs and along your shins for a slimming hint of shimmer. Bonus: This delicious-smelling product is actually good for your skin. It's packed with antioxidant-rich nutrients and vitamins that have been known to deliver anti-aging and skin-restorative benefits.

And while 80 percent of 1,500 men surveyed by *Men's Health* answered that they're more into butts and breasts than legs, let's not forget about your stems, either. If you're still fretting about them after your first 6 weeks of the program, it's time to streamline them too! To do so, you're going to increase the weight you've been using and really challenge them, says LBN workout designer Rachel Cosgrove. "Do not be afraid of bulking up!" she says. "You have to put a demand on your body that it's not accustomed to in order for it to change."

The exercises in this chapter will do much more than break your habit of exiting a room backside first. They'll also ease your back pain, improve your balance, and make it easier for you to move more gracefully through your day even in those mundane moments of everyday life.

CUSTOMIZED LEG AND BUTT WORKOUT

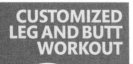

phase 3: WEEKS 7 TO 9

instructions: Perform 2 to 3 sets of 6 to 8 reps with 60 seconds of rest between exercises. Use a weight that's heavy enough to make any additional reps nearly impossible without a breather.

leg and butt circuit

EXERCISE	SETS	REPS	TEMPO/TIME	REST
2A: Single-Leg Squat*	2-3	6-8/side	moderate	60 sec
2B: Romanian Deadlift with Barbell*	2-3	6-8	moderate	60 sec
2C: Step up*	2-3	6-8/side	moderate	60 sec
2D: Hip-Flexor Stretch	2-3	1/side	30 sec	60 sec

workout A

EXERCISES	SETS	REPS	TEMPO/TIME	REST
Dynamic Warmup	See page 106			
Circuit 1:				
1A: Plank on Swiss Ball	1-2	1	60–90 sec	60 sec
1B: Core Stability Twist*	1-2	15	moderate	60 sec
Circuit 2:				
Customized Leg and Butt Circuit				
Circuit 3:				
3A: Hip Extension	2-3	6-8	moderate	60 sec
3B: One-Point Dumbbell Row*	2-3	6-8/side	moderate	60 sec
3C: Front Squat*	2-3	6-8	moderate	60 sec
3D: Single-Arm Dumbbell Chest Press on a Swiss Ball*	2-3	6-8/side	moderate	60 sec

workout B

EXERCISES	SETS	REPS	TEMPO/TIME	REST
Dynamic Warmup	See page 106			
Circuit 1:				
1A: Prone Jackknife	1-2	10–15/side	moderate	60 sec
1B: Prone Cobra on a Swiss Ball	1-2	1	60–90 sec	60 sec
Circuit 2:				
Customized Leg and Butt Circuit				
Circuit 3:				
3A: Split Squat with Opposite Arm Overhead Press*	2-3	6-8/side	moderate	60 sec
3B: Wide-Grip Pulldown*	2-3	6-8	moderate	60 sec
3C: Single-Leg, Single-Arm Romanian Deadlift*	2-3	6-8/side	moderate	60 sec
3D: Inverted Row	2-3	6-8	moderate	60 sec

* Add weight as you progress in the program.

2A
single-leg squat

start

- Stand on your left leg. Extend your right leg so that the heel is just off the floor. Raise your arms in front of you so that they're parallel with the floor.

movement

- Bend the supporting knee and lower your body as far as you can. Keep your left foot flat on the floor and your back straight.

- Take 3 seconds to reach the bottom of the movement, and then immediately explode back to the starting position. Your range will be limited at first, but try to increase it as you improve. (Increase your number of reps, too, but your range is just as important, if not more so.)

- If you can exceed 15 reps using only your own body weight, hold a dumbbell in your right hand, but keep it at your side.

Tip

You may hold a squat rack with one hand for balance, but do not use it to pull yourself up.

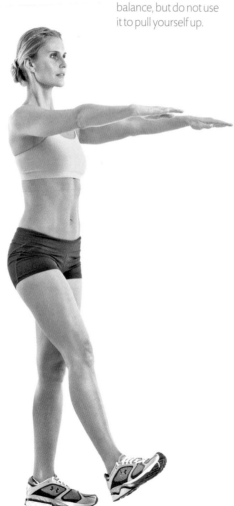

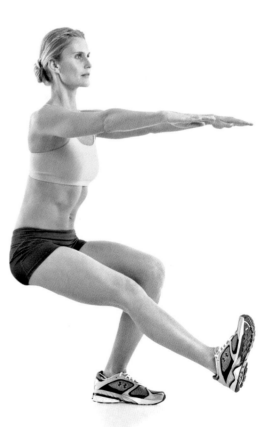

2B
romanian deadlift with barbell

start

* Stand holding a barbell in front of your thighs with an overhand grip. Your feet should be shoulder-width apart with your feet flat on the ground. Bend your knees slightly.

movement

* Push your hips back a few inches. Keeping your back straight, bend at the waist and begin lowering your torso toward the floor. Lower the barbell toward the floor as you descend, keeping the bar as close to your body as you can. You'll feel a stretch in your hamstrings.

* Go as low as you can, pause for a moment, and then slowly return to the starting position and repeat.

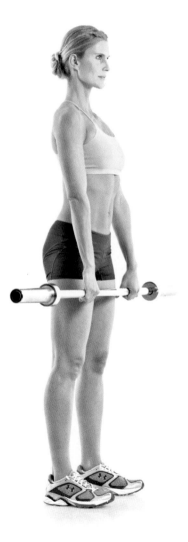
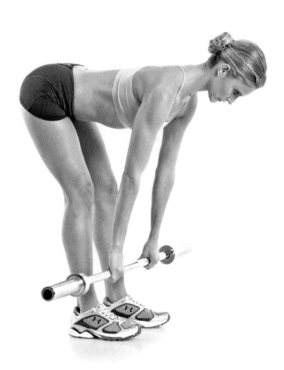

3A

stepup

start
• Stand facing a low step. Place your left foot on it.

movement
• Push through your left foot and lift your body up. Your right foot will leave the floor, but do not allow it to touch the bench. Lower yourself to the floor under control, pause briefly, and repeat. Be sure to use only your left leg; do not bounce and push off your right. Complete all reps with your left leg before repeating with your right.

Tip
For an added challenge, increase the height of the step—eventually you'll want to use a bench. Then add load in the form of dumbbells.

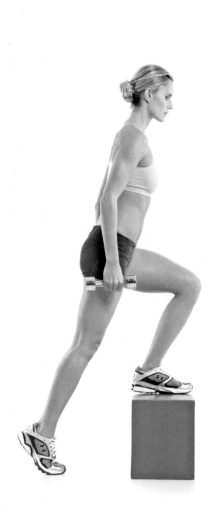
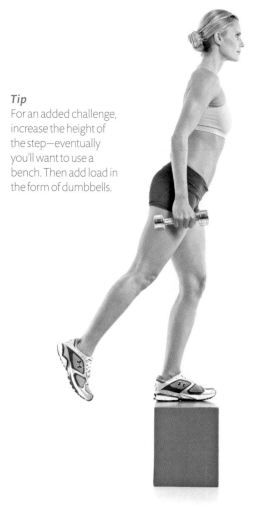

2D
hip-flexor stretch

start

- Kneel on your right knee, your left foot flat on the floor. Keep your torso upright and rest your hands on your left knee.

movement

- Gently push your hips forward while keeping your torso upright. You should feel a stretch in the front of your right hip. Hold the stretch for 60 seconds, switch legs, and repeat.

- To intensify the stretch, turn your body away from your back leg. You can also raise your right arm straight over your head and lean away from your back leg.

Tip

For a different version of this exercise, stand facing away from a bench. Place your right foot on the bench and lower into a lunge, as if you were doing a Split Squat (see page 000), but then lean forward to feel the stretch in the front of your hip.

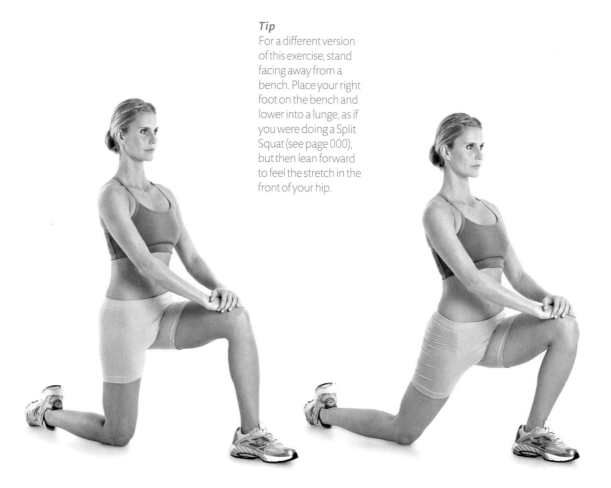

Blasting Cellulite

What works—and doesn't—to erase those dreaded ripples, bumps, and lumps

▶ Orange peel, cottage cheese—there's nothing pretty about cellulite or its nicknames. For many women it's private enemy number one. Nearly 82 percent of the 3,500 *Women's Health* readers who responded to my Look Better Naked survey cited cellulite as a potential barrier to baring all. Half of them were taking their lumps but weren't happy about it; the other half stated emphatically: "I want it gone ASAP."

Alas. Despite the myriad miracle "cures" for cellulite making the info-mercial rounds, there are no quick fixes. Even liposuction can't budge it. There are, however, a number of ways you can make it less noticeable. To help you understand how these measures work (and why other "treatments" don't), let's understand what cellulite actually is. Basically, it's just plain old subcutaneous fat—meaning just beneath the skin—that has a

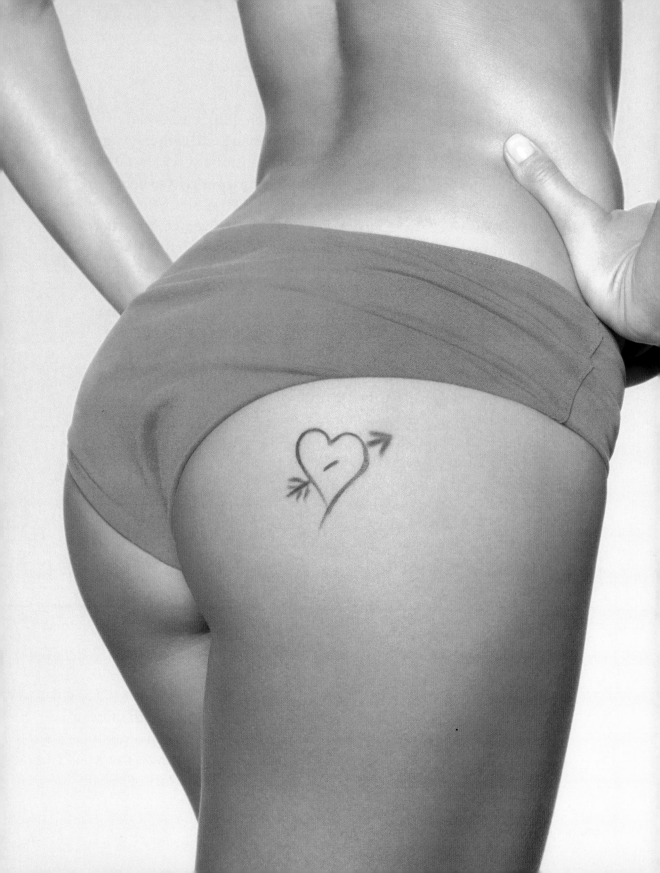

puckered texture, according to Alexander J. Koch, PhD, an associate professor of health and exercise sciences at Truman State University in Kirksville, Missouri. In areas where you see cellulite, however, the fat (along with water and lymph, the clear fluid that carries cells to help fight infections and other diseases throughout the body) is pushing through a mesh of fibrous bands that connect skin to muscle. In women, these fibers form a honeycomb pattern, so any increase of fat tends to bulge. Imagine squeezing a fishnet stocking over a water balloon—that's basically what's going on with cellulite.

Experts don't know exactly what causes cellulite, but they believe that genes, hormones, and, of course, excess fat are to blame. Regardless of what causes it, cellulite is a bigger problem for women than for men. In fact, it really doesn't affect men at all. For one thing, guys naturally carry around less fat than we do. But they also don't retain fluids as easily as women; they produce much, much less estrogen; and their connective tissue doesn't form the same weblike pattern as ours.

It's small consolation that this is a problem that can just as easily affect a movie star as it can you. According to the Mayo Clinic, at least 8 in 10 women have some cellulite. In addition to the moves in this chapter, here are some ways you can counter the ripple effect.

Hard-Body Hardware

In 2007, researchers in Lincoln, Nebraska, set out to learn which cardio machines kick your butt the hardest. So long as you're jogging instead of walking on a treadmill, you'll activate 48.9 percent of your gluteus maximus, according to their study. Keep that in mind when you're in need of an activity on your do-anything day!

Fry Excess Fat

The less mush you have, the less mush there is to poke up through those annoying fibers. But here's the thing: You have to cut calories in order to cut fat. "Studies have proven that exercise alone, without changes to the diet, will not substantially reduce weight or body fat," says Koch. The LBN diet was structured with calorie intake in mind. If you're serious about combating cellulite, follow the eating plan for 3 additional weeks—simply mix and match your favorite meals—while also using the fitness strategy in this chapter.

Do Interval Training

As an adjunct to diet, interval training—like what you've been doing during your metabolic workouts—is the best way to incinerate subcutaneous fat. "Claims that specific exercises, like jumping rope or weight training, will somehow target cellulite aren't well documented at all," explains Koch. "What research has shown is that high-intensity interval training is more effective in reducing subcutaneous fat than is performing lower-intensity work." For example, a study from Canada found that exercisers who did 30-minute workouts that included short, hard efforts lost three times as much fat in 15 weeks as their peers who performed steady-paced, easier workouts for 45 minutes. "Technically, you burn more fat as fuel during low-intensity exercise," says researcher Jason Talanian, PhD, who did a series of studies on interval training at the University of Guelph in Ontario. "But you become a better fat burner overall [even when resting] by raising your fitness ceiling, which you do by going fast." Specifically, Talanian found that interval training increases your cells' fat-frying ability by up to 50 percent. And because interval workouts are harder to do than pokey one-speed workouts, your body takes longer to return to normal after you're done—meaning you keep torching calories long after you've showered.

Rub It In, Rub It In

Certain creams that claim to smooth cellulite may temporarily do so. They usually contain caffeine to stimulate bloodflow and help flush excess fluids. To get the best results from a product such as St. Ives's Cellulite Shield Gel Crème ($8, at drugstores), slather a thick body lotion over it to help the ingredients penetrate better after you've applied it to your skin.

Camouflage Your Ripples

Dimples will seem to melt into a hint of tan, but be careful how you bronze. I recommend getting your color from a self-tanner. If you opt to tan the all-natural way—at the beach for instance—protect yourself by using La Roche-Posay Anthelios SPF 40 sunscreen ($32, laroche-posay. us). It provides complete protection from UVA and UVB rays, and contains Mexoryl SX, a compound that won't degrade quickly in sunlight.

What you should avoid at all costs are tanning beds. In an analysis of 20 studies recently published in the medical journal *The Lancet Oncology*, researchers came to a scary conclusion: Your skin cancer risk increases by

Zen Bump Zappers

▶▶ Some yoga enthusiasts swear by inversion poses for purging puckery skin, claiming that these upside-down positions move lymph along. Here are two that may iron out dimples. If you're new to the yoga mat, have an instructor help guide you through the poses—then do them every other day.

Modified shoulder stand
Lie on your back with your arms by your sides. Bend your knees and rock your legs up, bringing your knees to your forehead and placing your hands under your hips to support them. Keeping your elbows on the floor, hold for 8 to 10 breaths. Then slowly release your knees and roll gently back onto the mat.

Plow pose
Begin in the modified shoulder stand. Straighten your legs, extending them back out over your head, and rest your toes on the floor. Straighten your arms on the floor, palms down. Hold for 8 to 10 breaths before bending your knees back to your forehead and lowering your body down onto the mat.

75 percent if you use tanning beds before age 30. Experts have also moved tanning beds and ultraviolet radiation from "probable carcinogens" into the highest cancer risk category: "carcinogenic to humans." Other members of that group include arsenic, tobacco, and mustard gas.

As I said, I prefer self-tanners, and I learned a few helpful pointers from Meredith Baraf, the makeup artist who gets the Victoria's Secret models perfectly faux-bronzed.

• *Exfoliate.* For even results, it's a must. Baraf recommends using a fine-grained scrub like Mark's Costa Rica Body Smoothing Exfoliator ($10, meetmark.com). It sloughs with bamboo-stem extract and walnut-shell powder. Rub a palmful of scrub all over your body in a circular motion, concentrating on rough spots such as elbows and knees (where self-tanner can get blotchy), then rinse off.

• *Moisturize.* Choose a body lotion with a gradual self-tanner. "Moisturizing first helps the tanning product go on more smoothly. Using one with a mild bronzing agent does the additional job of disguising any spots you may miss," Baraf says. Try Hawaiian Tropic Island Glow Daily Moisturizer ($7, at drugstores). Let this layer dry for 10 to 15 minutes before you apply self-tanner or bronzer.

• *Mist on bronzer.* Experts recommend sprays over creams: "They go on evenly and don't require rubbing, which causes streaks," says Baraf. Try L'Oréal Paris Pro Perfect Airbrush Self-Tanning Mist ($10, drug store. com). Hold the can a foot away from your body and spray in a circular motion. "Start with your legs—if you bend down to do them with wet tanner on your top half, you'll wind up with creases," she warns. And skip your ankles and feet, since the gradual tanner mentioned above will provide enough color there. From your legs, move up to your torso, neck, arms, and back (you might need help from a friend for that part).

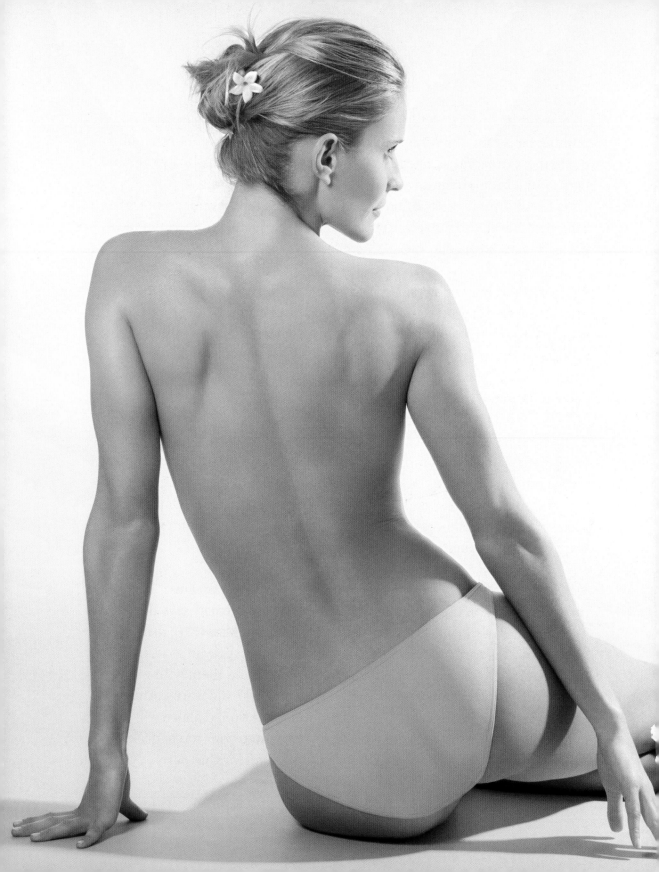

sculpted shoulders, toned arms

The secret to a firm upper body

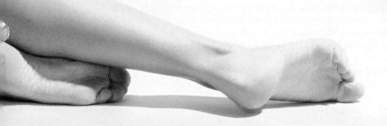

Your eyes may be the window to your soul, but your arms and shoulders are a window to the rest of your body. Besides your face, they're the parts you display most often and bare most readily—in T-shirts and tank tops as well as in sleeveless dresses and strapless gowns. That high-stakes visibility makes them the de facto barometer of the state of your shape. If your biceps are gracefully contoured, if the backs of your arms are firm and strong, if your shoulders are square and lifted, then the casual observer will assume that the rest of you is just as fit and toned. And they'll probably be right, because if you're like the majority of women, you've put more into toning your lower body than your upper body. "Women tend to be all about losing fat, and levels of body fat tend to be perceived as a bigger problem than puny arms," says Keli Roberts, a trainer in Pasadena, California, and co-author of *Stronger Legs and Lower Body*. My survey of *Women's Health* readers bears this out: Only about 23 percent of respondents said their "supporting cast" needed more attention than their "leading roles."

But I'm here to tell you that you can get just as much LBN mileage out of shaping your shoulders and sculpting your arms as you can from flattening your belly. Case in point: The attention Michelle Obama has received for showing off her awesome arms. The most elegant first lady since Jackie O. appeared sleeveless at 10 inaugural balls, at her husband's address to Congress, and in her official White House portrait. Google "Michelle Obama's arms" and you'll get 1,510,000 results—from debates about whether such "exposure" is appropriate for a FLOTUS (evidently it's inappropriate for a woman to display her dedication to a healthy lifestyle) to speculation about her routine. That latter piece of information was so coveted that you'd think it was deemed top secret . . . until *Women's Health* declassified it! (Learn more on page 283.)

Of course, having arms and shoulders you can display proudly isn't going to land you in the White House, but consider these compelling payoffs:

Square Your Shoulders

Stand with your back, shoulder blades, and hips against a wall. Place the backs of your raised arms and hands against the wall. (Your elbows should be bent at 90 degrees, with your upper arms parallel to the floor.) Slowly straighten your elbows while sliding your arms up into a V. Then slowly return to the starting position. Repeat to complete 2 sets of 10 reps.

You'll Look More Feminine!

There's generally not a lot of fat around a woman's deltoids, so muscle growth there is more defined under your skin, according to Lou Schuler, co-author of *The New Rules of Lifting for Women.* So not only will these exercises provide some instant gratification, they'll also build bolder shoulders—which will accentuate an hourglass-shaped figure by making your waist appear smaller!

You'll Have a Stunning Fashion Accessory!

Formal events such as weddings have a dress code for a reason: You need to look good—not just for the big day but for Facebook and the photo books, too. But you'll probably need to show some arm because so many designers

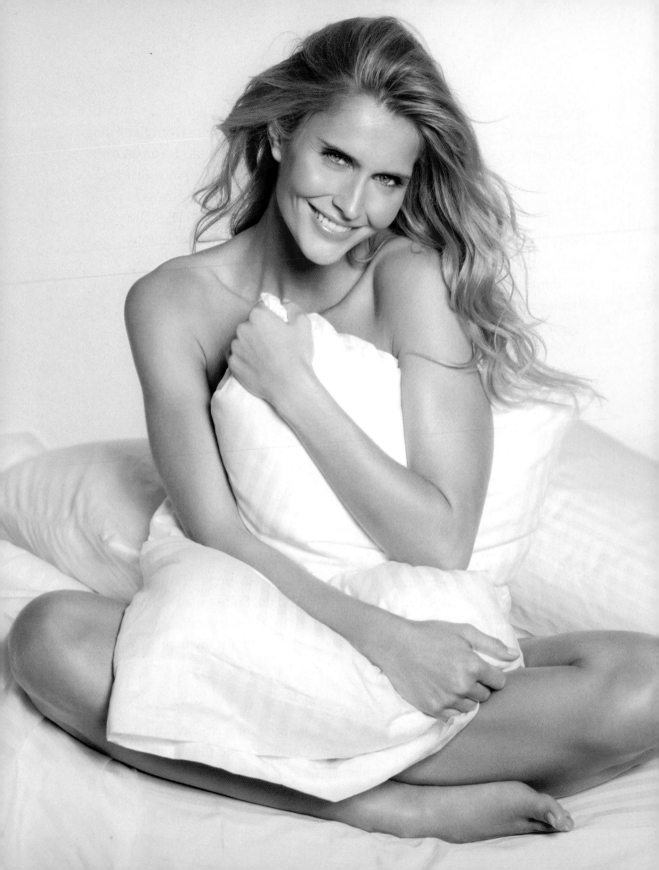

have embraced strapless and sleeveless dresses in recent years. Which is a good thing, in my opinion, because a beautiful pair of shoulders and arms can rival a glittering necklace. So just imagine what they'll do for your confidence when you're away from all your pretty dresses and wearing a bikini or even just a post-shower towel!

You'll Prevent Injuries!

Letting your spine sag—all too easy when you're spending endless hours in front of a computer and then lounging around when you get home— causes imbalances, forcing the muscles and ligaments in your neck, shoulders, back, and legs to compensate. What's more, we use the muscles in the front of our shoulders more than those in the back, and as they tighten our posture tends to tilt forward. This, of course, makes you more prone to injuries, such as sharp pains between your shoulder blades or a chronic feeling of tightness in your upper back—especially after you've lugged

Who's Got the Best Arms of All?

In my survey of 3,500 women, Michelle Obama walked away the hands-down winner for BEST ARMS. However, the first lady focuses on much more than her arms during her thrice-weekly workouts—which reportedly take place at 5:30 a.m. The foundation of her workout, designed by her longtime trainer, Cornell McClellan, is an intense weight-training routine made up of compound movements that work multiple muscle groups. In one session, Mrs. Obama might do 1 set of 15 to 20 reps each of lunges, bench presses, hip raises, and rows, all without resting—and with short bouts of intense cardio mixed in. For an even greater total-body challenge, her workouts also feature jumping rope, kickboxing, and body-weight calisthenics, all done at a heart-and-lung-busting pace that skyrockets fitness levels and burns tons of calories. The result: a woman who's earned the right to be a health and fitness role model because she knows firsthand just how much dedication it takes to make it a lifestyle.

around overstuffed grocery, shopping, or diaper bags. Finally you'll be able to shoulder these items without struggling!

The arms and shoulder circuit LBN workout designer Rachel Cosgrove created for this chapter primarily targets the muscles that get called on for all these challenges—the biceps and triceps of the upper arms as well as the latissmus dorsi and main deltoid (or shoulder) muscles. But to maximize calorie burn, Cosgrove selected exercises that work more than one group of muscles at a time. The result is a more efficient workout that doesn't waste your time by isolating individual muscles and that sculpts as it strengthens. Prepare for some instant gratification: Because there's relatively less fat on the upper body compared with the lower body, it's impossible to obscure the results of weight training. You're going to see the results of your effort *fast*!

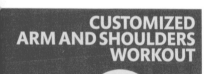

CUSTOMIZED ARM AND SHOULDERS WORKOUT

phase 3: WEEKS 7 TO 9

instructions: Perform 2-3 sets or 12 reps each, resting 30 seconds between most exercises.

arm and shoulders circuit

EXERCISE	SETS	REPS	TEMPO/TIME	REST
2A: Close-Grip Pulldown*	2-3	12	moderate	30 sec
2B: Lateral Raise with External Rotation*	2-3	12	moderate	30 sec
2C: Incline Dumbbell Chest Press*	2-3	12	moderate	30 sec
2D: Chest Stretch	2-3	1/side	30 sec	30 sec

workout A

EXERCISES	SETS	REPS	TEMPO/TIME	REST
Dynamic Warmup	See page 106			
Circuit 1:				
1A: Plank on Swiss Ball	1-2	1	60–90 sec	60 sec
1B: Core Stability Twist*	1-2	15	moderate	60 sec
Circuit 2:				
Customized Arms and Shoulders Circuit				
Circuit 3:				
3A: Hip Extension	2-3	12	moderate	30 sec
3B: One-Point Dumbbell Row*	2-3	12/side	moderate	30 sec
3C: Front Squat*	2-3	12	moderate	30 sec
3D: Single-Arm Dumbbell Chest Press on a Swiss Ball*	2-3	12/side	moderate	30 sec

workout B

EXERCISE	SETS	REPS	TEMPO/TIME	REST
Dynamic Warmup	See page 106			
Circuit 1:				
1A: Prone Jackknife	1-2	10–15/side	moderate	60 sec
1B: Prone Cobra on a Swiss Ball	1-2	1	60–90 sec	60 sec
Circuit 2:				
Customized Arms and Shoulders Circuit				
Ciruit 3:				
3A: Split Squat with Opposite Arm Overhead Press*	2-3	12/side	moderate	30 sec
3B: Wide-Grip Pulldown*	2-3	12	moderate	30 sec
3C: Single-Leg, Single-Arm Romanian Deadlift*	2-3	12/side	moderate	30 sec
3D: Inverted Row	2-3	12	moderate	30 sec

* Add weight as you progress in the program.

2A
close-grip pulldown

start

• Sit at a pulldown machine. (You can also kneel on a pad at a pulley machine, which is preferable because it keeps your hips in extension.) Grab the bar or handles with an overhand grip, with your hands about shoulder-width apart.

movement

• Pull the bar down. (It helps if you think about pulling your chest upward.) Bring your elbows to your sides and the bar to your chest, and then slowly return to the starting position.

Tip

To make the exercise more challenging, do chinups instead to recruit more of your core muscles. Hang from a chinup bar with your palms facing you. Pull yourself upward until your chin clears the bar, then return to the starting position. You can start by using a band for assistance. The band, which wraps over the bar and can extend as low as your knees, supports your body as you're lifiting yourself. The thicker the band, the easier the chinup will be.

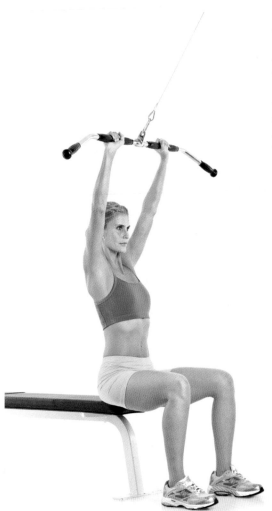
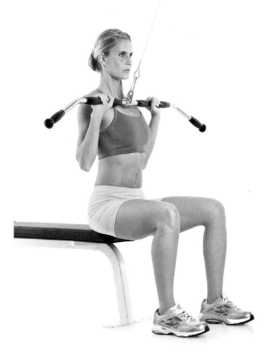

lateral raise with external rotation

start

- Stand with your feet shoulder-width apart. Hold a dumbbell in each hand alongside your body. Bend your elbows 90 degrees, so that the weights are in front of and slightly beneath your chest.

movement

- Maintaining the L shape of your arms, raise your elbows out at your sides until your upper arms are parallel to the floor and your forearms point straight down.

- Keeping your elbows level with your shoulders and keeping your wrists in line with your forearms, rotate your upper arms to raise the dumbbells in an arc until they're directly above your elbows. Reverse the movement and return to the starting position.

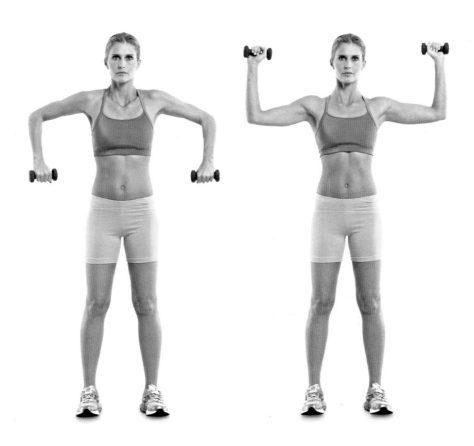

2Cw
incline dumbbell bench press

start

- Lie on your back on an incline bench and hold a dumbbell in each hand. Place the weights alongside your chest about 8 to 10 inches away from your body, with your palms facing your feet.

movement

- Push the dumbbells straight up until your arms are fully extended. The dumbbells should nearly touch in this top position. Lower them to the starting position.

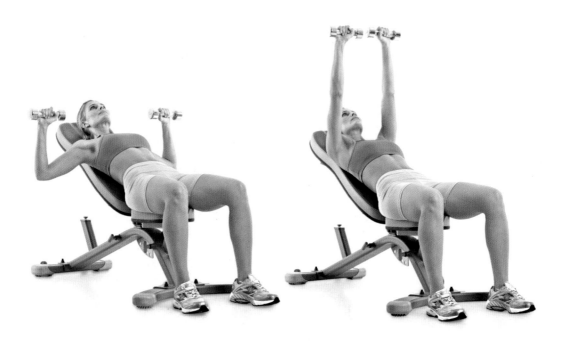

2D
chest stretch

position

• With your palm and forearm firmly against a wall or doorway and your elbow at a 90-degree angle, walk or lean your torso away from that point to stretch your chest. Repeat on the opposite side.

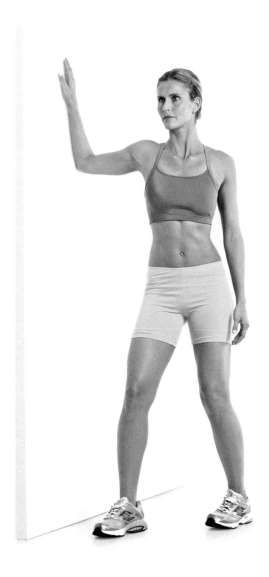

Tip

For an alternate version, lie on a foam roller, positioned so that it's beneath your spine and also supports your head. Relax your arms at your sides until you begin to feel a stretch in your chest. Bend your elbows at a 90-degree angle and try raising them slightly to increase the stretch even more.

The Road Warrior
Upper-Body Workout

When you can't get your hands on a set of dumbbells, your body weight will do in a pinch. Use it to maintain your LBN workout results with this sequence of exercises created by Jessica Matthews, a certified personal trainer with the American Council on Exercise in San Diego. It focuses on the arms and shoulders but also includes core and leg moves for strength and support. For best results, complete one circuit of all the exercises two to three times per week.

Pushup

Get into a pushup position. Slowly lower your body toward the floor, then press up until your arms are fully extended. During the entire exercise, keep your head aligned with your spine, and don't allow your lower back to sag or your hips to hike up. Do 8 to 12 reps.

Make it harder: Lift your left foot off the floor, keeping your leg extended throughout the pushup. Return to the starting position and repeat with your right leg elevated. Alternate legs as you complete the set. Do 8 to 12 reps.

Downward-Facing Dog

From a pushup position with your arms and legs fully extended (wrists directly under shoulders), contract your core and abdominal muscles. Slowly exhale and shift your weight backward by pushing your hips up and back. Continue moving until your body forms an inverted V, allowing your head to hang loosely between your shoulders. Keep your arms and legs extended, and be sure to maintain a neutral (flat) spine. Hold for 1 to 2 minutes.

Make it harder: From downward-facing dog, move forward into a plank position (the top of a pushup) and pull your right knee toward your chest, engaging your core as you bring your knee in. Press back to downward-facing dog as you place your right foot back on the floor. Repeat with your left leg. Do 8 to 12 reps per side.

Side Plank

Lie on your left side with your legs extended, your left elbow directly under your shoulder, and your right hand palm resting on your right hip. Stack your right foot on top of your left. As you exhale, gently contract your abs and lift your hips and knees off the floor, keeping the side of your left foot and your left forearm and elbow in contact with the floor. Hold for 15 to 30 seconds. Switch sides and repeat.

Make it harder: Raise your top leg off your supporting leg throughout the exercise.

Opposite-Limb Raise

Lie on your stomach with your arms extended overhead, palms facing each other, and your head and neck in line with your spine. As you exhale, contract your abs to stabilize your torso and slowly raise one leg and the opposite arm a few inches off the floor simultaneously. Hold this position briefly before returning to the starting position. Alternate sides with each rep. Don't arch your back or bend your neck. Do 8 to 12 reps.

Make it harder: Raise both arms and both legs off the floor. Hold briefly, then gently inhale and lower your legs and arms back to the floor without creating any movement in your lower back or hips.

Plankup

Starting in the plank position, lower onto your forearms keeping your elbows under your shoulders. Keep your abs tight and your back straight. Hold for 5 seconds, then extend your left arm straight out in front of you. Lower your left arm back down to the forearm plank position and repeat with your right arm. That's 1 rep. Do 8 to 12 reps.

Make it harder: No need: This one's tough enough as is!

Credits

Cover and Chapter Openers

Pages: 1, 7, 10-11, 14, 18-19, 45, 93, 103, 167, 179, 191, 197, 225, 245, 263, 273, 278-279, 282

Photographs by Ondrea Barbe

Styling: Thea Palad
Prop Styling: Manny Norena
Hair: Robert Lyon for Kerastase Paris at Atelier Management
Makeup: Samantha Trinh for Dior Beauty at Atelier Management
Manicurist: Nausil Zaheer/ Mark Edward Inc.

Fitness

Photographs by Beth Bischoff
Styling: Thea Palad
Hair and Makeup: Michiko Boorberg
Pages: 3, 107-137, 144-161, 206-223, 232-235, 252-255, 268-271, 286-289

Meals

Photographs by Thomas MacDonald/Rodale Images
Food Stylist: Melissa Reiss
Photo Editing: Tara Long
Pages: 3, 51, 62, 65, 69-91, 194

Food

Photographs by Mitch Mandel/Rodale Images
Photo Editing: Tara Long
Pages: 55, 59, 61, 63, 64, 67

Inside Credits

index

h

Hair
    body acne and, 173
    hirsutism, 178
    ingrown, 184–85
Hair removal
    laser, 185
    shaving, 176–80
    sugaring, 181
    waxing, 181–85
Hammertoe, 189
HDL cholesterol, 61
Headaches, from cramped neck
    muscles, 249
Health club
    buying a membership,
        100–101
    credentials of instructors, 100
    location, 100
Health foods, 243
Heart disease
    lowering risk with
        exercise, 163
        flat abs, 229
    visceral fat linked to, 12, 17
Heels, exfoliating, 188
High blood pressure, decreased
    risk with fat abs, 229
Hip extension, 119, **119**, 208, **208**
Hip flexors, tight, 139, 228
Hip-flexor stretch, 235, **235**,
    271, **271**
Hirsutism, 178
Honey, 65
Horizontal wood chop on a
    Swiss ball, 234, **234**
Humectants, 170
Hummus, 58
Hunger, thirst confused with, 243

i

Imbalances. *See* Muscle
    imbalances
Implant, breast, 246
Incline dumbbell bench press,
    288, **288**

Incline pushup, 123, **123**
Ingrown hair, 184–85
Ingrown toenail, 189
Injury prevention
    with strong abdominal
        muscles, 229
    with toned upper body, 283–84
Insulin, 238
Internal obliques, 227
Interval training. *See also*
        Metabolic workout
    benefits of, 96
    conventional aerobic workout
        compared, 96
    for subcutaneous fat loss, 275
Inverted row, 217, **217**
Iron, 54, 55
Isometric exercise, 228
Italian spice mix, 63
Iyengar yoga, 27

j

Jojoba oil, 186
Journal, 240
Jumping rope, 137
Jump squat, 135, **135**
Junk food, 243

k

Keratosis pilaris, 176
Ketchup, 65
Kidney cancer, 229
Knees, rough skin on, 175

l

Laser hair removal, 185
Lateral jump, 109, **109**
Lateral pushup shuffle, 115, **115**
Lateral raise
    with external rotation, 287, **287**
    standing alternating, 131, **131**
Lava rock, 188
Legs
    bronzer stick use, 265

    exercises
        hip-flexor stretch, 271, **271**
        Romanian deadlift, 269, **269**
        single-leg squat, 268, **268**
        stepup, 270, **270**
    shaving, 176–80
    waxing, 181–85
    workout
        circuit, 266
        exercises, 268–71, **268–71**
        workout A, 267
        workout B, 267
Letter to body part, writing, 21
Lightening cream, 170
Lighting
    for nude photograph, 41
    skin tone appearance and, 24
Lignans, 58
Lines, minimizing fine skin, 169
Lingerie, 38
Liposuction, 272
Lips, 170
Loincloth, 23
Longevity, 229
Lunch
    in LBN 2-day cleanse, 67
    in LBN 6-week diet
        week 1, 68–71
        week 2, 72–75
        week 3, 76–79
        week 4, 80–83
        week 5, 84–87
        week 6, 88–91
Lunge
    antirotation reverse, 232, **232**
    front-foot-elevated, 145, **145**
    stationary, 122, **122**, 137, **137**
Lunge walk with rotation and
    overhead reach, 113, **113**
Lycopene, 54

m

Makeup, 203
Mango salsa, 65
Marinade, yogurt-based, 64
Marinara sauce, 65
Massage, 37
Meals
    in LBN 2-day cleanse, 67